A Complete

Mediterranean

Cookbook

DISCLAIMER

No part of this eBook can be transmitted or reproduced in any form including print, electronic, photocopying, scanning, mechanical, or recording without prior written permission from the author.

While the author has taken utmost efforts to ensure the accuracy of the written content, all readers are advised to follow information mentioned herein at their own risk. The author cannot be held responsible for any personal or commercial damage caused by misinterpretation of information.

All information, ideas, and guidelines presented here are for educational purposes only and readers are encouraged to seek professional advice when needed

Are you looking for healthy recipes?

Do you want an easier and active lifestyle where cooking is minimal but nutritious?

Well you do not have to search anymore. This e-book includes just what you are looking for a healthier lifestyle. You do not have to worry about calories or boring food anymore. We have compiled for you a list of healthy, easy to make, nutritious recipes, which will provide you with just the lifestyle you are looking for.

This e-book introduces you to 50 Mediterranean recipes. Mediterranean recipes are known to lower the risk of heart diseases and other health problems, giving you just the healthy life you have always wanted!

Here is a glimpse of what you will find in this e-book

- 50 Mediterranean recipes
- Recipes to quickly put together for breakfast
- Recipes for meals including soups
- Recipes for healthy yummy salads
- Complete recipes with servings, cooking time, and nutritional information
- A systematic process for cooking so you know exactly what you need and how to proceed with the recipe

So, what are you waiting for? Read on to start your journey to a healthier life!

Contents

BREAKFAST RECIPES

Chorizo Scrambled Eggs

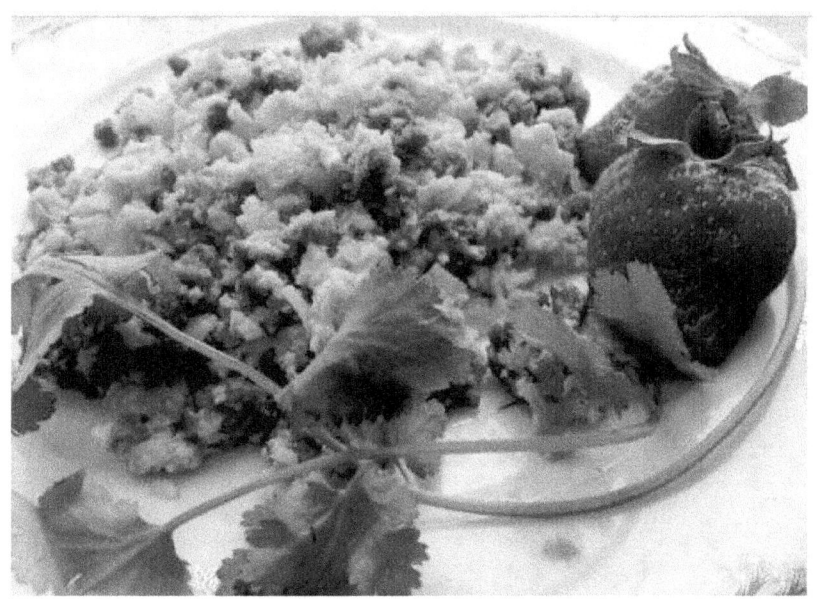

SERVINGS

2 persons

COOKING TIME

15-20 minutes

INGREDIENTS

Coconut oil: 1 tbsp

Diced onion: ½

Diced red pepper: 1

Sliced chorizo: ½ lb

Eggs: 4

Sea salt: a dash

Black pepper: ¼ tsp

PREPARATION METHOD

1. Sauté onions in coconut oil for 5 minutes in pa, over medium heat
2. Add chorizo and red peppers until crispy
3. Beat eggs with sea salt and pepper meanwhile
4. Pour into pan and scramble softly until cooked
5. Serve hot.

NUTRITION VALUE PER SERVING

Calories: 286

Fat: 14.3g

Protein: 34.8g

Carbohydrates: 9.1g

Zucchini Breakfast

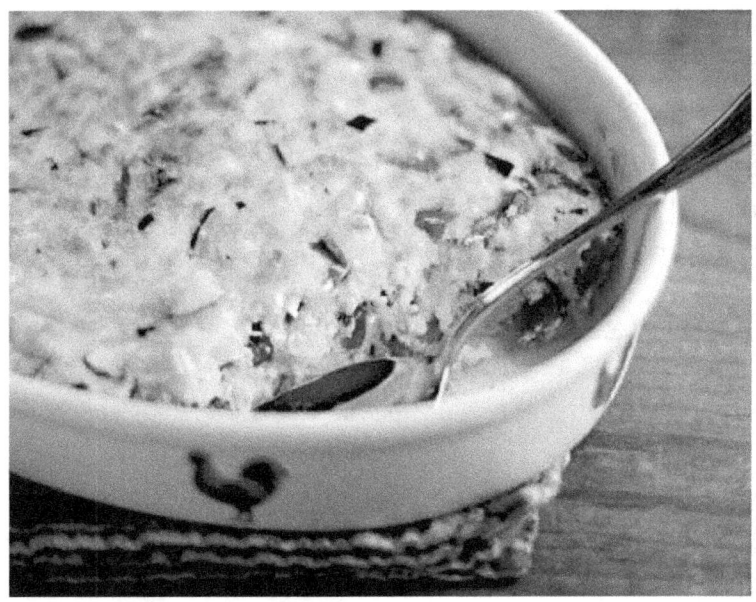

SERVINGS

4 persons

COOKING TIME

10-15 minutes

INGREDIENTS

Coconut oil: 2 tbsp

Chopped onion: 1

Shredded zucchinis: 4

Chopped tomatoes: 1 cup

Chopped garlic cloves: 2

Spinach: 2 cups

Sliced chicken sausage links: 2

PREPARATION METHOD

1. Cook chicken sausage in oil over medium heat (about 3 minutes).
2. Add and cook onion, garlic, zucchini and tomatoes (about 5 minutes) and then add spinach.
3. Place in plates and serve.

NUTRITION VALUE PER SERVING

Calories: 140

Fat: 10.8

Protein: 2.4g

Carbohydrates: 11.1g

Peachy Smoothie

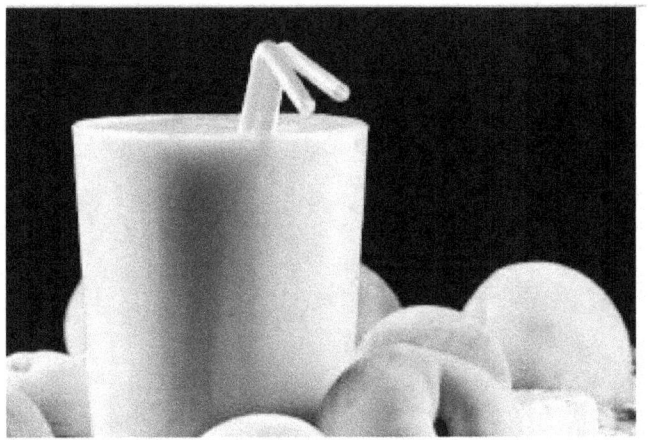

SERVINGS

2 persons

COOKING TIME

10 minutes

INGREDIENTS

Sliced banana: 1

Peeled orange: 1

Peach: 1

Coconut milk: 1 cup

Ice cubes: 4

Cinnamon: ½ tsp

Nutmeg: ½ tsp

Ginger: 1 tsp

Turmeric: 1tsp

Water: (as needed)

PREPARATION METHOD

1. Mix all ingredients in blender until smooth
2. Divide in two glasses and serve chilled.

NUTRITION VALUE PER SERVING

Calories: 400

Fat: 29g

Protein: 5g

Carbohydrates: 38g

Broccoli and Bacon Omelet

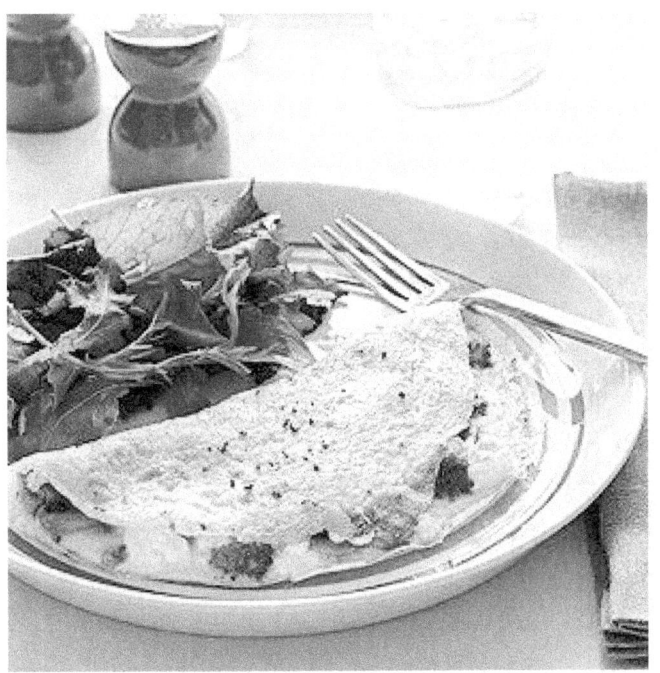

SERVINGS

2 persons

COOKING TIME

15-20 minutes

INGREDIENTS

Bacon slices: 4

Coconut oil: 1 tbsp

Diced onion: 1

Minced garlic cloves: 2

Chopped broccoli: 2 cups

Beaten eggs: 5

PREPARATION METHOD

1. Cook bacon on medium heat until crispy (5-8 minutes)
2. Cook diced onion in the meantime in other pan (3-4 minutes) and then add broccoli, cook until it becomes soft.
3. Add in garlic to bacon and cook for about 5 minutes. Stirring occasionally.
4. Cook eggs on both sides, place bacon slices and broccoli mixture over eggs. Fold and cut into two halves with spatula.
5. Serve with bread.

NUTRITION VALUE PER SERVING

Calories: 250

Fat: 18g

Protein: 20g

Carbohydrates: 11g

Breakfast smoothie

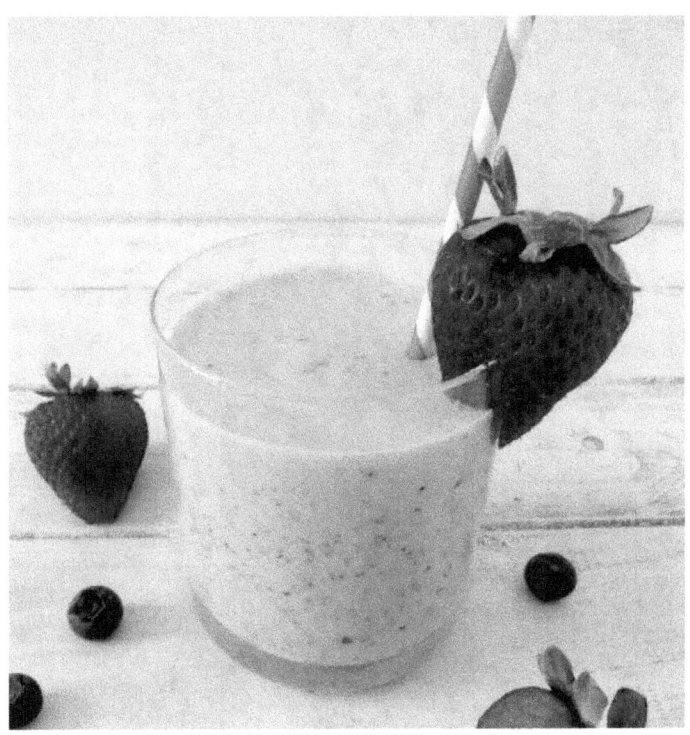

SERVINGS

2 persons

COOKING TIME

10 minutes

INGREDIENTS

Berries: 2 cups

Unsweetened shredded coconut: 2/3 cups

Almond milk: 1 cup

Eggs: 1-2

PREPARATION METHOD

1. Blend all ingredients together until smooth

2. Serve chilled.

NUTRITION VALUE PER SERVING

Calories: 380

Fat: 31g

Protein: 6.5g

Carbohydrates: 23g

Pancakes

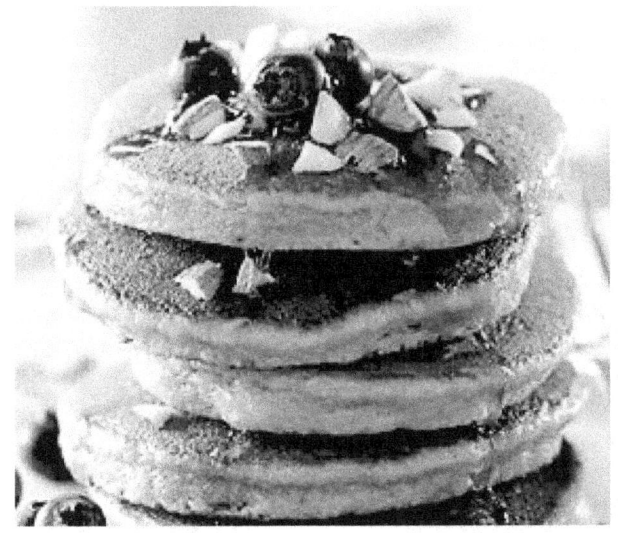

SERVINGS

4 persons

COOKING TIME

15-20 minutes

INGREDIENTS

Coconut flour: ¼ cup

Eggs: 3

Baking soda: ¼ tsp

Cinnamon: ½ tsp

Sea salt: ¼ tsp

Pumpkin puree: ¼ cup

Apple cider vinegar: ½ tsp

Coconut oil: 1 tbsp

Almond milk: ¼ cup

Maple syrup: ¼ cup

PREPARATION METHOD

1. Whisk the dry ingredients together.
2. Whisk the dry ingredients namely, eggs, coconut oil, apple cider vinegar, pumpkin puree and maple syrup in separate bowl.
3. Add dry mix to wet mix slowly, and combine well.
4. Heat pan over medium heat with coconut oil. Spoon batter into pan and keep an eye until done. Flip over when golden brown
5. Serve fresh and warm with maple syrup.

NUTRITION VALUE PER SERVING

Calories: 169

Fat: 10.3g

Protein: 4.7g

Carbohydrates: 15.9g

Mini Pizzas

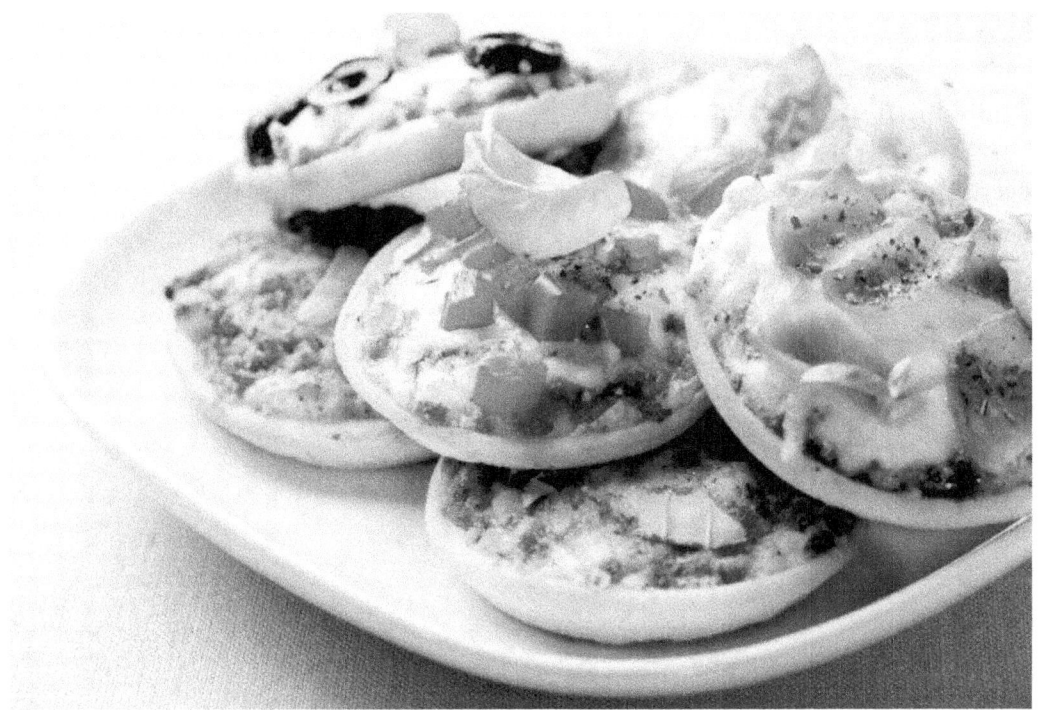

SERVINGS

4 persons

COOKING TIME

15 minutes

INGREDIENTS

English muffins: 2

Split eggs: 4

Pizza sauce: 1/3 cup

Shredded Italian cheese: ½ cup

Dried oregano

PREPARATION METHOD

1. Toast the muffin halves.
2. Preheat oven to 450 degree F.
3. Over medium heat, cook beaten eggs in coconut oil forming soft large curds.
4. Spread pizza sauce on muffins, lay egg and cheese, and bake for about 5-10 minutes.
5. Serve sprinkled with oregano.

NUTRITION VALUE PER SERVING

Calories: 198

Fat: 9g

Protein: 13g

Carbohydrates: 16g

Egg and Veggie Breakfast

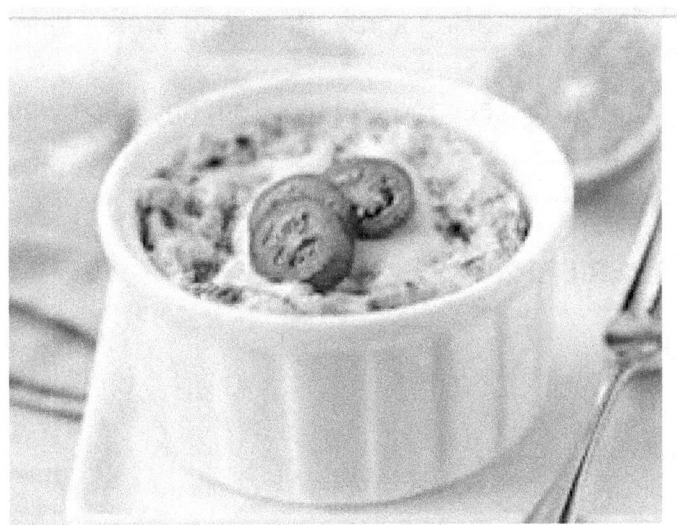

SERVINGS

1 person

COOKING TIME

5 minutes

INGREDIENTS

Egg: 1

Water: 1 tbsp

Thinly sliced baby spinach: 2 tbsp

Chopped mushrooms: 2 tbsp

Mozzarella cheese: shredded

Cherry tomatoes: sliced

PREPARATION METHOD

1. Coat custard cups with cooking spray. Beat, egg, water, spinach and mushrooms until blended.
2. Microwave mixture for 30 seconds on high, stir and microwave again for 30 seconds.
3. Serve with cheese and tomatoes on top.

NUTRITION VALUE PER SERVING

Calories: 100

Fat: 2g

Protein: 9g

Carbohydrates: 2g

Avocado Deviled Eggs

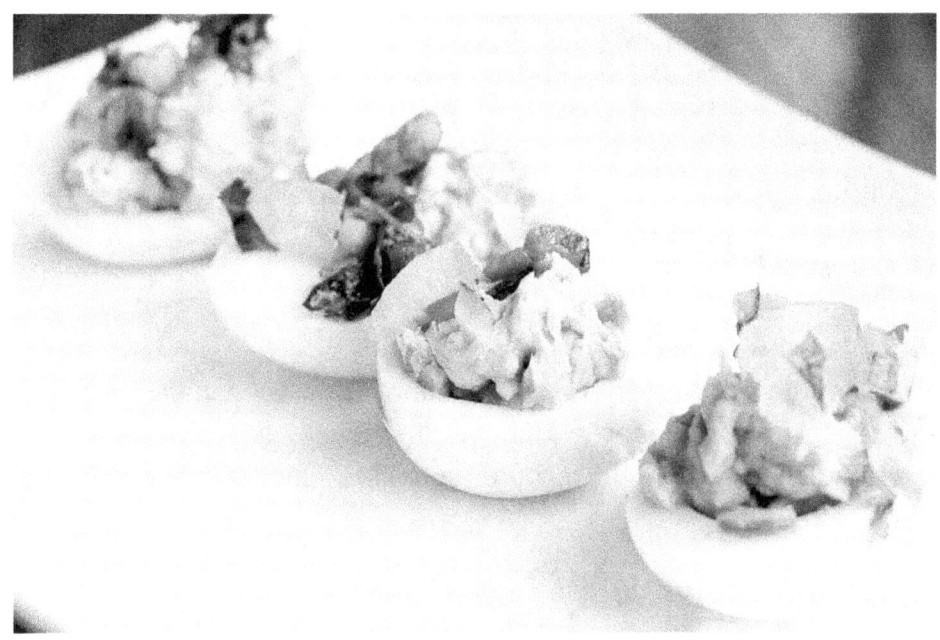

SERVINGS

8 persons

COOKING TIME

20-25 minutes

INGREDIENTS

Hard boiled, peeled eggs: 12

Peeled avocado: 1

Mayonnaise: ¼ cup

Ground cumin: 1 tbsp

Finely chopped capers: 1 tbsp

Dijon mustard: 1 tbsp

Juiced lemon: 1

Sea salt: ½ tsp

Chopped jalapeno peppers: 2

Chili powder: 1 tbsp

Chopped cilantro: 2 tbsp

PREPARATION METHOD

1. Cut eggs lengthwise and slip the yolks out.
2. Mash yolks with avocado in a bowl. Add mayonnaise, cumin, capers, mustard, lime juice, salt, and jalapeno and mix well.
3. Fill the egg white halves with mixture, sprinkle with cilantro and chili powder and it is ready to serve.

NUTRITION VALUE PER SERVING

Calories: 150

Fat: 14g

Protein: 7g

Carbohydrates: 2g

Strawberry Banana Smoothie

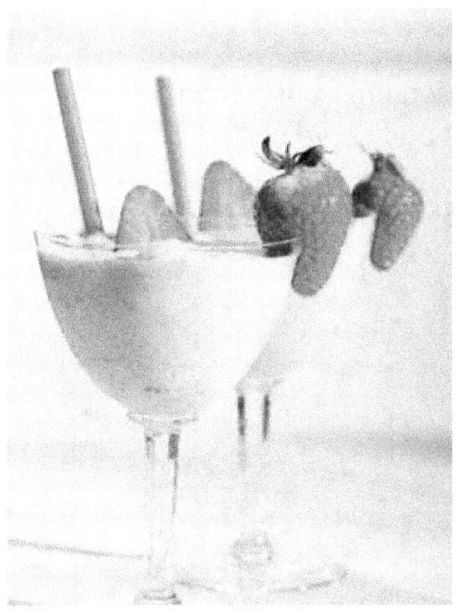

SERVINGS

2 persons

COOKING TIME

10 minutes

INGREDIENTS

Banana: 1

Sliced strawberries: ¾ cup

Fat-free yogurt: 1 ¼ cup

Skim milk: 1 ¼ cup

Orange juice: 2 tbsp

Flaxseed oil: 1 tbsp

Ice cubes

PREPARATION METHOD

1. Blend all ingredients together until smooth.
2. Divide in two glasses and serve chilled.

NUTRITION VALUE PER SERVING

Calories: 330

Fat: 8g

Protein: 17g

Carbohydrates: 48g

MEALS

Lamb Burgers

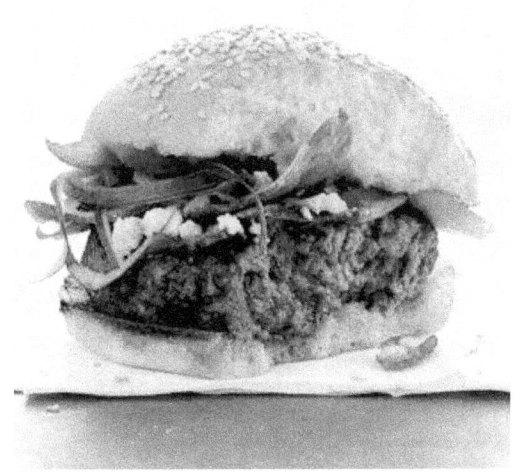

SERVINGS

2 persons

COOKING TIME

30 minutes

INGREDIENTS

Ranch lamb patties: 1 packet

Sweet potato (medium): 1

Romaine lettuce: 1(chopped)

Goat cheese

Chives

Mushrooms: 2

PREPARATION METHOD

1. Boil sweet potatoes until cooked
2. Thoroughly cook lamb patties over medium heat
3. Sauté mushrooms until soft and season with salt and pepper
4. Stack mushrooms on top of the chopped lettuce. Add sweet potatoes, lamb patty, goat cheese, and chives. Serve warm

NUTRITION VALUE PER SERVING

Calories: 103

Fat: 0.2g

Protein: 2.3g

Carbohydrates: 23.6g

Halibut with Artichoke and Olives

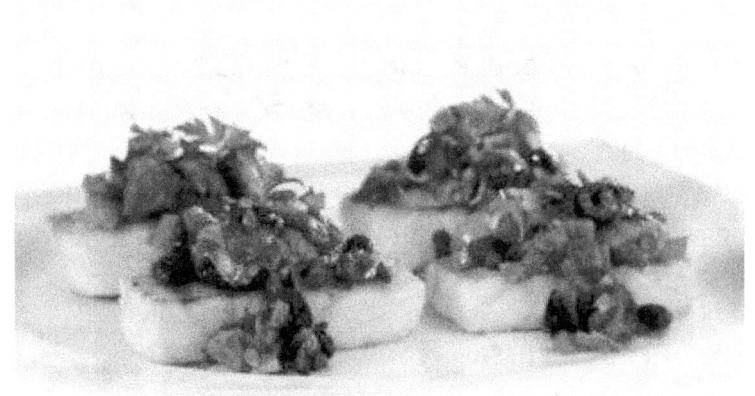

SERVINGS

4 persons

COOKING TIME

30 minutes

INGREDIENTS

Toasted pine nuts: ¼ cup

Halibut fillets: 4

Pepper and sea salt: according to taste

Grass fed butter: 3 tbsp

Lemon juice: ¼ cup

Crushed garlic clove: 1

Shredded fresh basil leaves: 5 tbsp

Kalamata olives: ½ cup

Frozen artichoke hearts: 1 cup

PREPARATION METHOD

1. Pre heat oven to 350 degrees
2. Season fish with salt and pepper and place in the baking dish
3. Melt butter with crushed garlic clove in a small saucepan. Add lemon juice and pour over the fish fillets
4. Top the fillet with olives and artichoke hearts
5. Bake for approximately 10-15 minutes by covering with aluminum foil
6. Serve with pine nuts and remaining fresh basil!

NUTRITION VALUE PER SERVING

Calories: 155

Fat: 15.4g

Protein: 1.4g

Carbohydrates: 1.9g

Pepper Steak

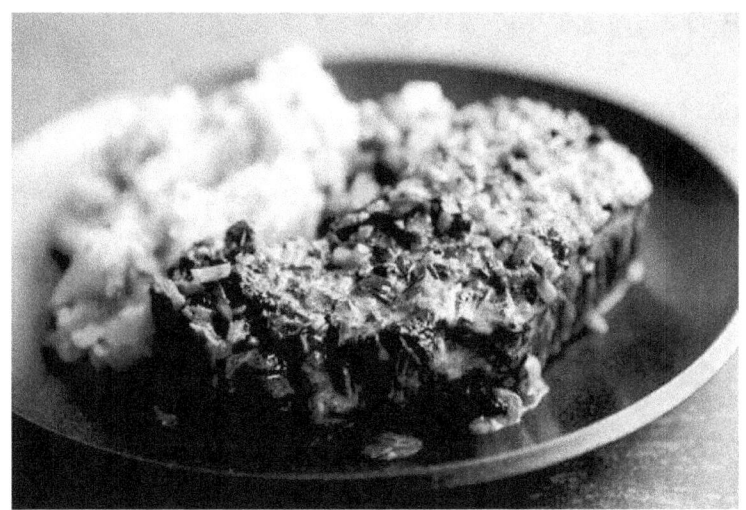

SERVINGS

2 persons

COOKING TIME

30 minutes

INGREDIENTS

Beef round steak: 1lb

Coconut oil: 2 tbsp

Sliced onion: 1

Sliced green pepper: 1

Water: ¼ cup

Garlic salt: ¼ tsp

Freshly ground black pepper for garnish

Shredded carrots: 4

PREPARATION METHOD

1. Cut stake into two slices
2. Brown meat and onions in skillet with oil over medium heat
3. Stir in water, green peppers and garlic salt and stir constantly for 5 minutes.
4. Serve hot with black pepper garnish on a bed of chopped carrots.

NUTRITION VALUE PER SERVING

Calories: 583

Fat: 20g

Protein: 74g

Carbohydrates: 22g

Mediterranean Chicken Pasta

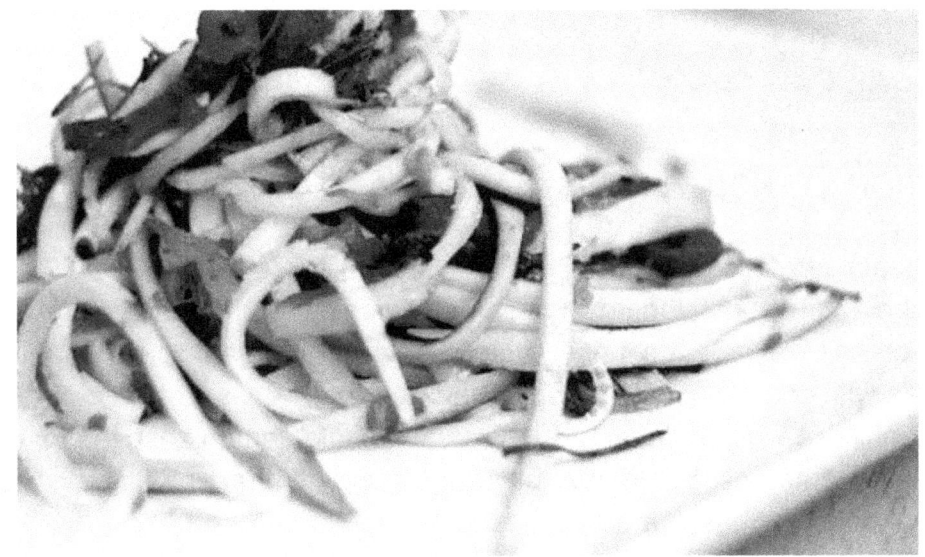

SERVINGS

4 persons

COOKING TIME

1 hour

INGREDIENTS

Chicken breast: 1 lb

Spaghetti squash: 1

Coconut oil: 2 tbsp

Sun-dried tomatoes: ½ cup

Can of black olives: 3.25 oz

Pine nuts: ¼ cup

Extra virgin olive oil: ¼ cup

Juice of ½ lemon

Salt and pepper: to taste

Garlic powder: 1 tsp

Basil

PREPARATION METHOD

1. Pre heat oven to 375 degree F
2. Put spaghetti squash length wise on baking sheet with water and bake for 1 hour
3. Season chicken breast chunks with salt, pepper and garlic powder and put in pan heated with coconut oil over medium heat.
4. Cook chicken well, and then add olives, pine nuts, lemon zest, lemon juice and sun dried tomatoes. Stir in olive oil after turning off heat and place mixture on top of spaghetti with basil garnish
5. Serve warm!

NUTRITION VALUE PER SERVING

Calories: 416

Fat: 29.3g

Protein: 37.9g

Carbohydrates: 2.4g

Fish Soup

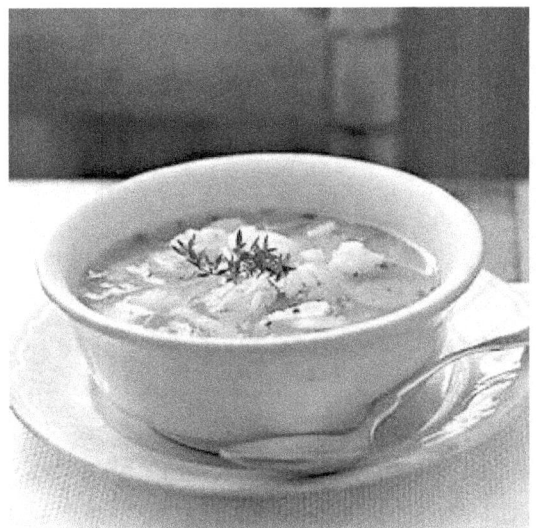

SERVINGS

6 persons

COOKING TIME

1 hour

INGREDIENTS

Coconut oil: 2 tbsp

Chopped onion: 1

Chopped garlic cloves: 3

Sliced tomatoes: 6

Bay leaf: 1

Fresh mint

Water: 8 cups

Small fish: 1 whole (cleaned and cut into 4 pieces)

Salt and pepper

Juiced lemon: 2

Fresh parsley

PREPARATION METHOD

1. Sauté onion and garlic until soft and golden in a large pot.
2. Bring mixture to boil after adding tomatoes, bay leaf, mint, and water. Reduce heat and add fish. Cook until soft.
3. Separate fish from soup, and remove its head, tail, skin, and bones.
4. Add cleaned fish to broth, and drizzle with lemon juice, salt, and pepper.
5. Serve hot with fresh mint and parsley.

NUTRITION VALUE PER SERVING

Calories: 190

Fat: 5g

Protein: 20g

Carbohydrates: 14g

Herbed Chicken and Spinach Soup

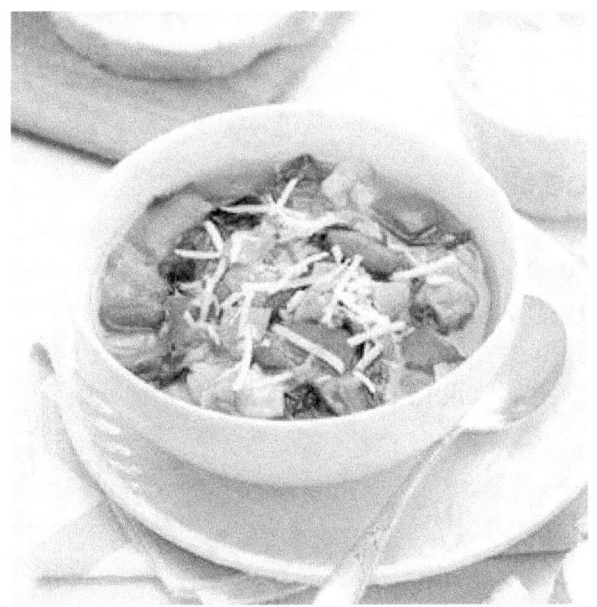

SERVINGS

6 persons

COOKING TIME

30-40 minutes

INGREDIENTS

Coconut oil: 1 tbsp

Boneless chicken breasts: 1 pound

Chopped carrots: 2 cups

Thinly sliced celery: 1 cup

Chopped onions: 1 cup

Dried thyme: 1 cup

Dry bay leaf: 1

Chicken stock: 4 cup

Dried parsley: 1 tbsp

Chopped spinach leaves: 1 cup

PREPARATION METHOD

1. Cook chicken in coconut oil on medium heat, stirring occasionally.
2. Add carrots, celery, onion, thyme and bay leaf, stirring until onion is soft.
3. Cook broth for 20-25 minutes in the mixture.
4. Stir in spinach, parsley, salt and pepper after removing from heat.
5. Serve warm

NUTRITION VALUE PER SERVING

Calories: 160

Fat: 4g

Protein: 21g

Carbohydrates: 10g

Grilled zucchini with lemon salt

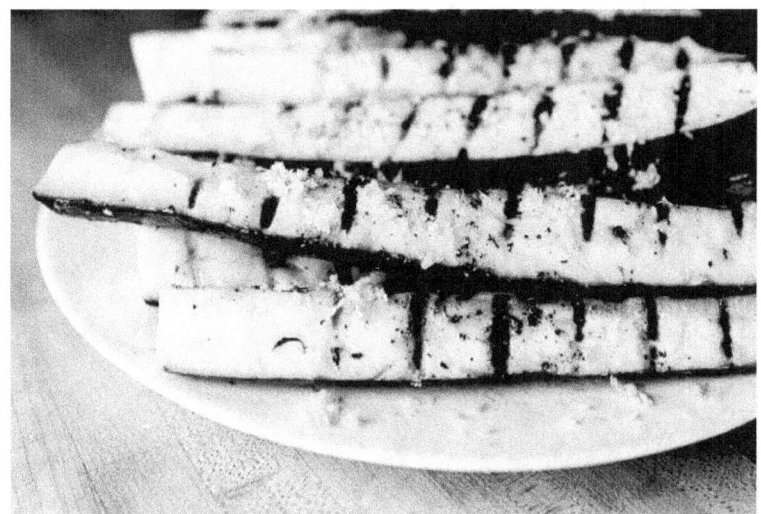

SERVINGS

8 persons

COOKING TIME

20-25 minutes

INGREDIENTS

Medium sized zucchini: 6

Extra virgin olive oil: ¼ cup

Kosher salt: 1 tsp

Black pepper: 1 tsp

Lemon zests: 3 whole

PREPARATION METHOD

1. Slice zucchinis into quarters lengthwise. Drizzle in olive oil, 1 tsp salt, pepper, 1 tbsp lemon zest and juice of two lemons over zucchinis in a plastic bag and seal it. Set aside to marinate for 20 minutes.
2. Prepare grill on medium heat and grill zucchinis on all three sides.

3. Sprinkle kosher salt on zucchinis in plate and serve.

NUTRITION VALUE PER SERVING

Calories: 55

Fat: 6.3g

Protein: 0g

Carbohydrates: 0.2g

Swiss Chard Stems With Tahini

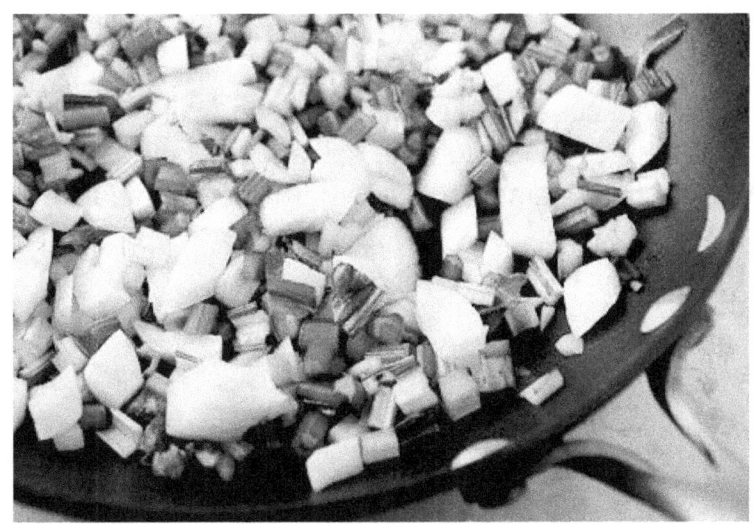

SERVINGS

4 persons

COOKING TIME

15 minutes

INGREDIENTS

Swiss chard: 1 bunch (only stems)

Tahini: ½ cup

Lemon juice: 2 tbsp

Water: 3 tbsp

Salt and pepper

Fresh parsley

PREPARATION METHOD

1. Cut chard stems into cubes and boil until tender. Drain and set aside.
2. Stir tahini, lemon juice, and water with salt and pepper to taste. Mix well.
3. Pour sauce over chard stems and serve garnished with parsley.

NUTRITION VALUE PER SERVING

Calories: 200

Fat: 16g

Protein: 7g

Carbohydrates: 11g

Chicken Stew with Peppers

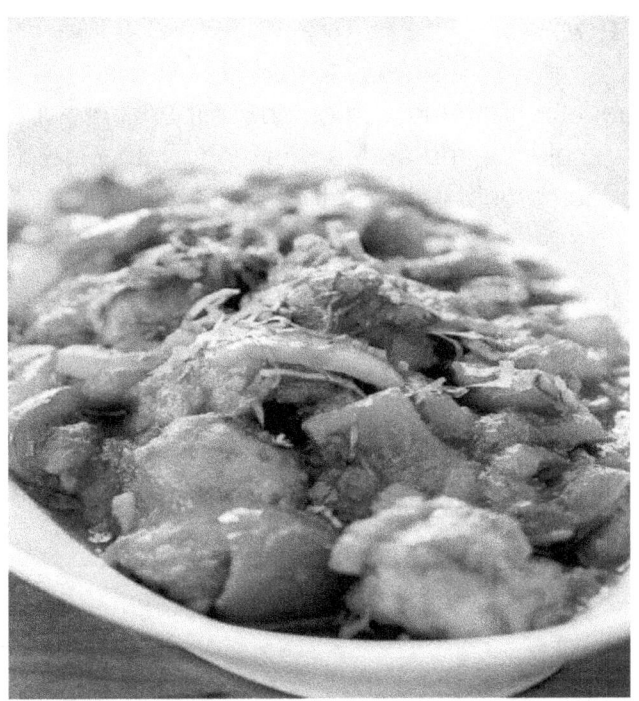

SERVINGS

8 persons

COOKING TIME

40 minutes

INGREDIENTS

Young chicken: 1

Coconut oil: 1 ½

Onion: 1 medium

Canned tomatoes: 1 cup

Sliced peppers: 1

Salt and pepper: to taste

PREPARATION METHOD

1. Heat oil over medium heat and add onions, stir until brown.
2. Cut chicken into 8 pieces and add to pan along with wine. After wine has evaporated, add tomatoes, pepper strips, salt and pepper. Cover and cook for 30 minutes.
3. Serve warm.

NUTRITION VALUE PER SERVING

Calories: 292

Fat: 6g

Protein: 9g

Carbohydrates: 6g

Cauliflower with Chickpeas

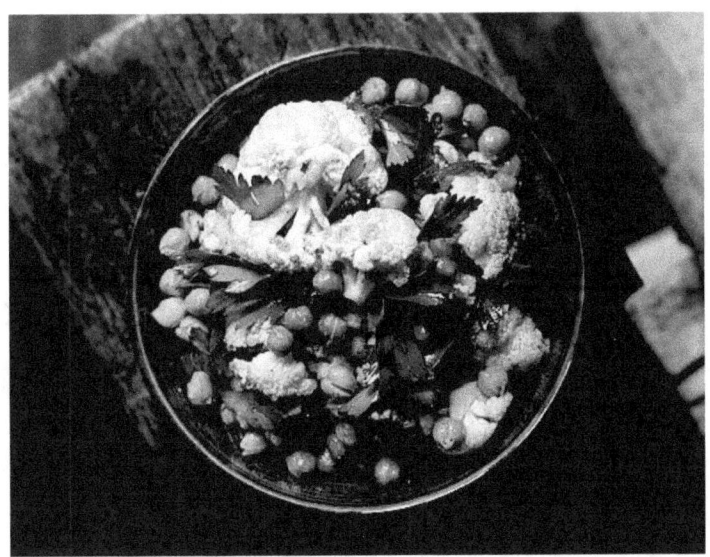

SERVINGS

4 persons

COOKING TIME

15 minutes

INGREDIENTS

Extra virgin coconut oil: 2 tbsp

Chopped onion: 1

Chopped yellow squash: 1

Chopped red pepper: 1

Cauliflower: 1

Cumin: 1 tsp

Diced tomatoes: 1 can

Chickpeas: 1 can

PREPARATION METHOD

1. Heat coconut oil and add onion, squash and pepper until vegetables soften.
2. Add cauliflower and sprinkle cumin. Cook for 5 minutes.
3. Stir in tomatoes and chickpeas and cook for 5 more minutes.
4. Serve immediately.

NUTRITION VALUE PER SERVING

Calories: 260

Fat: 1g

Protein: 9g

Carbohydrates: 40g

Honey Mustard Chicken

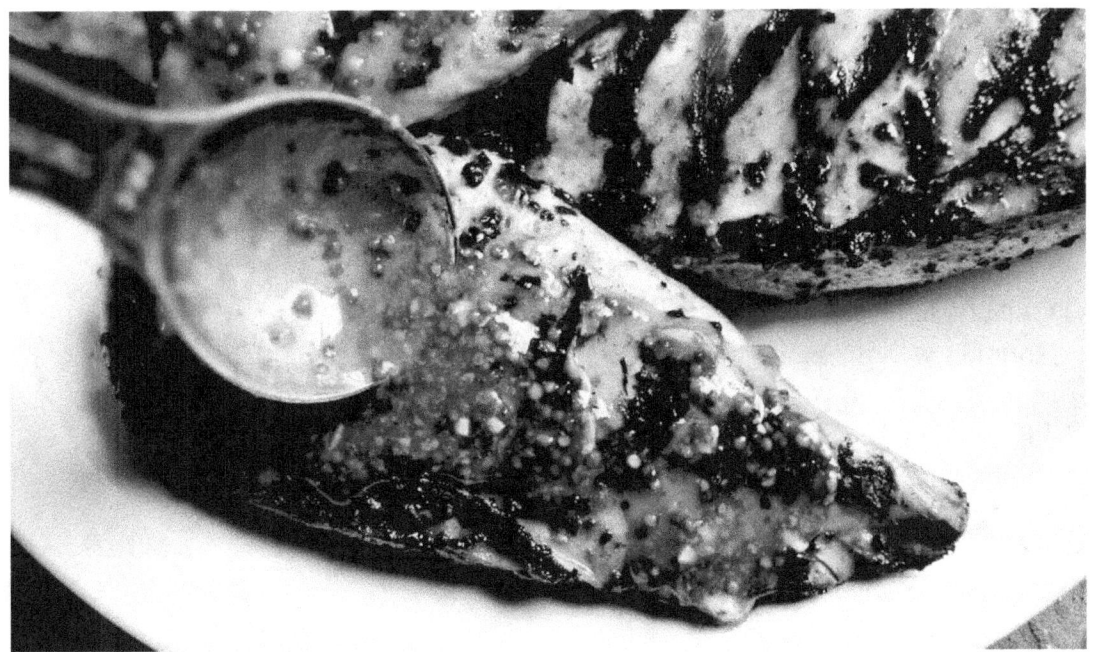

SERVINGS

6 persons

COOKING TIME

1 hour

INGREDIENTS

Boneless chicken breasts: 6

Chopped green onions: 2

Chopped parsley: 2 tbsp

For Marinade

Balsamic vinegar: 1/3 cup

Coconut oil: 2 tbsp

Honey mustard: ¼ cup

Crushed garlic clove: 1

Salt and pepper

PREPARATION METHOD

1. Make the marinade by combing all the ingredients in a bowl. Whisk well to combine. Pour the marine over chicken in shallow baking dish and allow to marinate.
2. Grill chicken on each side for about 5 minutes or until it is brown.
3. Sprinkle with green onions and serve hot.

NUTRITION VALUE PER SERVING

Calories: 277

Fat: 10g

Protein: 27g

Carbohydrates: 4g

Spaghetti

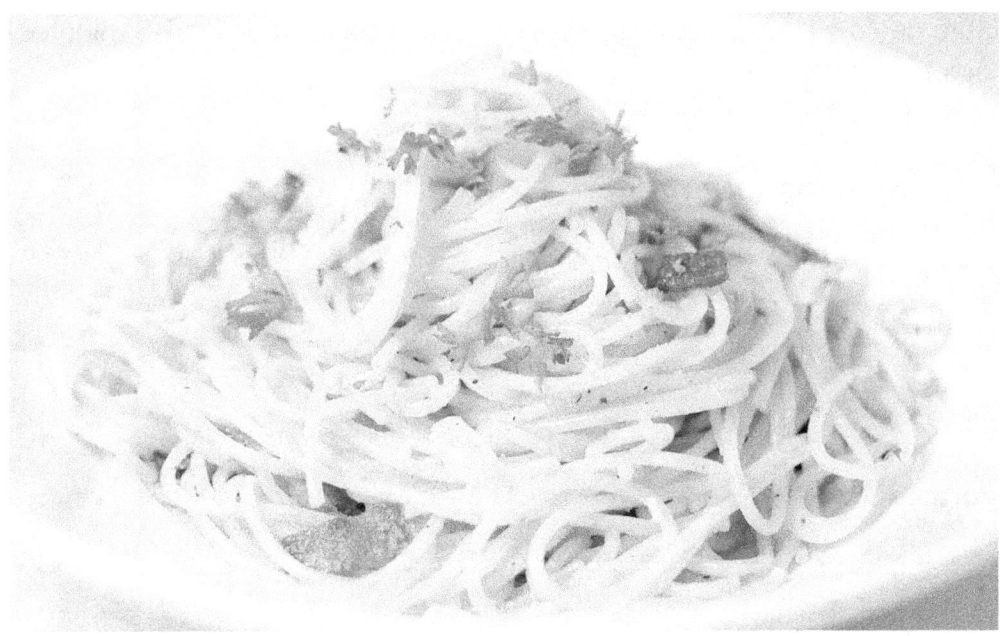

SERVINGS

8 persons

COOKING TIME

30 minutes

INGREDIENTS

Coconut oil: 1/3 cup

Minced garlic cloves: 3

Chopped parsley: 1/3 cup

Red chili pepper flakes: ¼ tsp

Grated parmesan cheese: ¼ cup

Whole-grain spaghetti: 1 box

PREPARATION METHOD

1. Sauté garlic, parsley and red pepper flakes in coconut oil for 2-3 minutes
2. Cook the pasta and add to the skillet.
3. Garnish with cheese and serve hot.

NUTRITION VALUE PER SERVING

Calories: 294

Fat: 3g

Protein: 8g

Carbohydrates: 43g

Spicy Chicken Patties

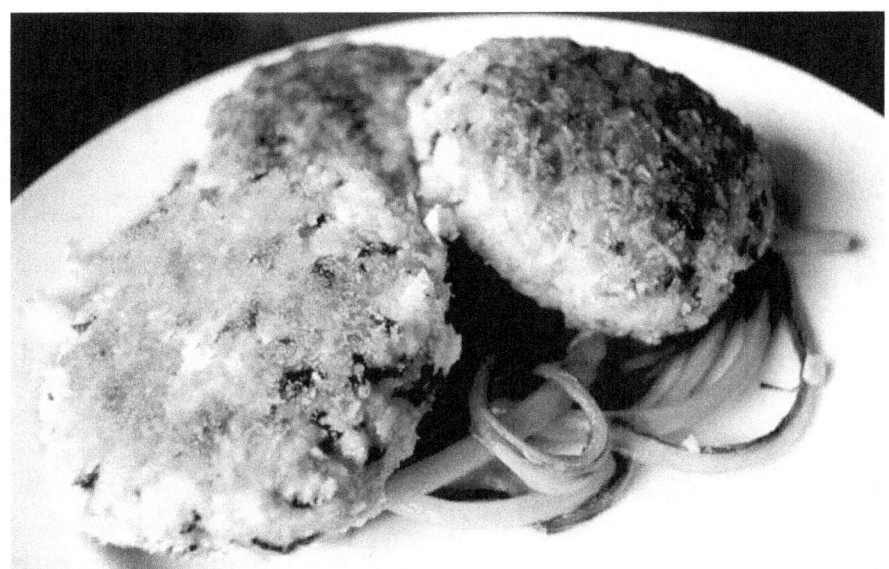

SERVINGS

6 persons

COOKING TIME

20 minutes

INGREDIENTS

Ground chicken: 1 pound

Egg: 1 large

Finely minced zucchini: ½

Finely chopped onion: ¼ cup

Chopped parsley: ¼ cup

Minced garlic: 1 tbsp

Salt: 1 tsp

Cayenne pepper: ½ tsp

Ground coriander: ½ tsp

Ground nutmeg: ¼ tsp

Ground cumin: ¼ tsp

Coconut oil: 3 tbsp

PREPARATION METHOD

1. Heat 1 tbsp oil in pan over medium heat and sauté zucchini for about 3 minutes.
2. Combine chicken, eggs, zucchini, onion, parsley, garlic, salt, and spices in a large bowl. Mix well with a fork.
3. Line baking sheet with foil and drizzle oil. Make 6 equal sized patties and place on baking sheet.
4. Broil for about 4-6 minutes or until lightly brown, flip and repeat.
5. Serve with tomato and cucumber on the sides.

NUTRITION VALUE PER SERVING

Calories: 81

Fat: 8g

Protein: 1.5g

Carbohydrates: 1.8g

Mediterranean Grilled Chicken

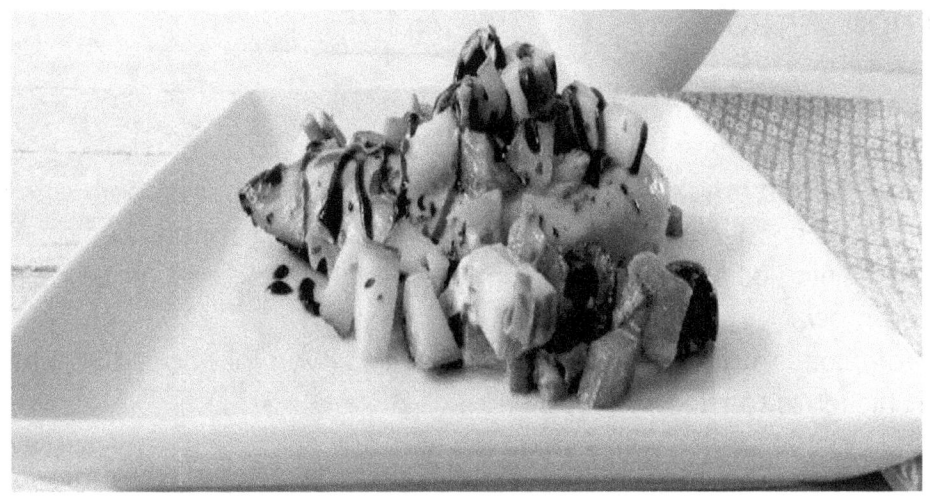

SERVINGS

2 persons

COOKING TIME

35 minutes

INGREDIENTS

Cherry or grape tomatoes: 1 cup

Pitted and halved kalamata olives: 18

Rinsed capers: 3 tbsp

Coconut oil: 2 tbsp

Boneless chicken breasts: 4

Sea salt

Ground pepper

PREPARATION METHOD

1. Pre heat oven to 475 F
2. In a bowl, toss tomatoes, olives, capers, and 2 tsp coconut oil.
3. Season chicken breasts with sea salt and ground pepper on both sides.
4. Add 2 tsp coconut oil on a skillet over high heat and sear chicken on both sides.
5. Add remaining oil and turn heat to medium-high. Cook until chicken breasts turn golden-brown.
6. Add tomatoes mixture to skillet and transfer to oven for about 15-18 minutes, until chicken is roasted through.
7. Serve in plates topped with tomato mixture!

NUTRITION VALUE PER SERVING

Calories: 631

Fat: 34.8g

Protein: 66.8g

Carbohydrates: 12.2g

Vegetable Kebabs Dipped In Yogurt Sauce

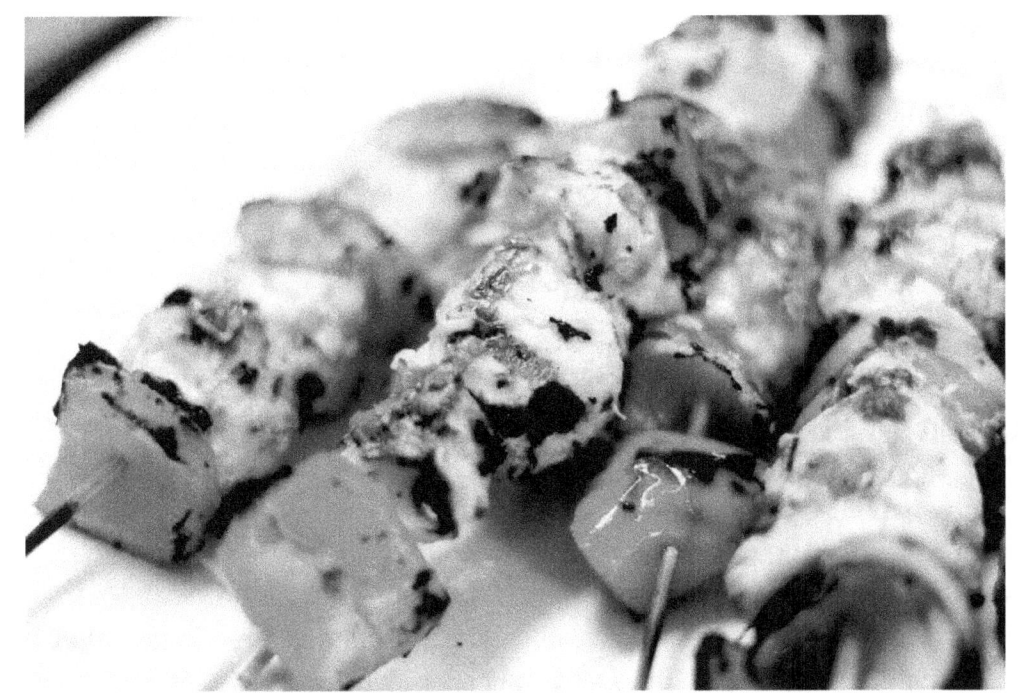

SERVINGS

4 persons

COOKING TIME

60-80 minutes

INGREDIENTS

Peeled and finely chopped cucumber: 1

Plain Greek yogurt: 1 ¼

Finely chopped onion: 1 tbsp

Finely chopped mint: 1 tbsp

Cherry tomatoes: 32

Sliced fresh corn cob: 1

Squared-cut yellow bell pepper: 1

Sliced zucchini: 2

Squared cut onion: 1

Coconut oil: 2 tbsp

Salt

Pepper

PREPARATION METHOD

1. Place cucumber in a colander, sprinkle with salt and pepper and allow to drain for 1 hour to make the sauce.
2. Add it in a bowl with yogurt, onion, and mint and refrigerate.
3. Thread vegetables onto skewer with kebabs brushed with oil and salt. Grill for 8 to 10 minutes, turning occasionally until slightly brown.
4. Serve warm with the sauce.

NUTRITION VALUE PER SERVING

Calories: 130

Fat: 7g

Protein: 8g

Carbohydrates: 10g

Soup with White Bean and Escarole

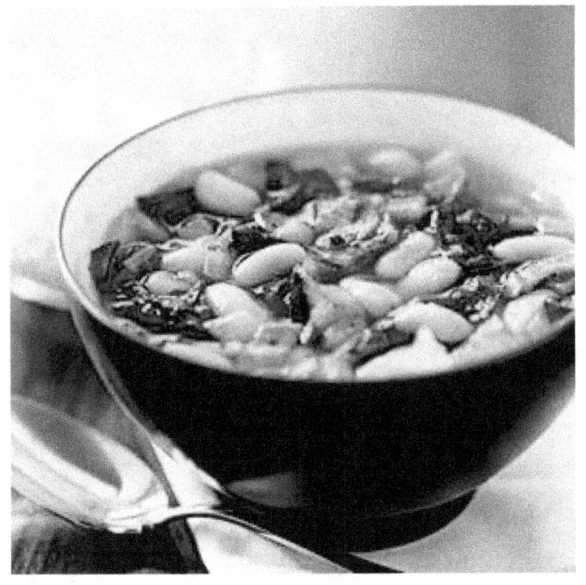

SERVINGS

4 persons

COOKING TIME

20-25 minutes

INGREDIENTS

Coconut oil: 1 tbsp

Chopped garlic cloves: 2

Peeled and chopped carrots: 3

Chopped onion: 1

Fresh parsley: 1/3 cup

Chopped pancetta: 1 oz

Chicken broth: 4 cup

Chopped escarole: 6 cups

Cannellini: 1 can

Parmesan cheese: grated

PREPARATION METHOD

1. Heat coconut oil over medium high heat. Add garlic, carrots, onion, parsley, and pancetta. Cook until brown for 4 minutes. Add the chicken broth and bring to boil
2. Reduce heat and add escarole and beans. Simmer for 10 to 15 minutes, stir occasionally.
3. Pour in bowls, topped with grated parmesan cheese and serve warm.

NUTRITION VALUE PER SERVING

Calories: 252

Fat: 5g

Protein: 14g

Carbohydrates: 41g

Mediterranean Styled Scallops with Zucchini

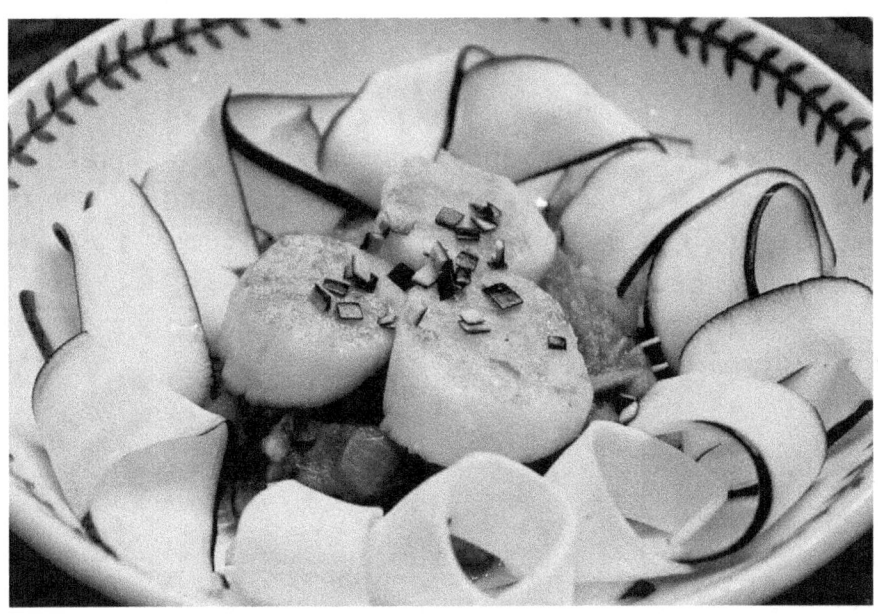

SERVINGS

2 persons

COOKING TIME

10-15 minutes

INGREDIENTS

Curry powder: 1 tsp

Ground ginger: ¼ tsp

Cumin: ½ tsp

Zucchini: 2

Squared cut bell peppers: 1

Sea scallops: 2 lbs

Coconut oil: 2 tbsp

Chopped fresh cilantro: ¼ cup

PREPARATION METHOD

1. Heat grill to medium and spray with cooking spray
2. Combine curry powder, ginger, and cumin in a small bowl. Thread scallops, zucchini and bell pepper onto skewers. Brush with oil and sprinkle spice mixture
3. Grill each side for 3 minutes or until golden
4. Serve hot sprinkled with cilantro.

NUTRITION VALUE PER SERVING

Calories: 215

Fat: 7g

Protein: 30g

Carbohydrates: 8g

Grilled Salmon

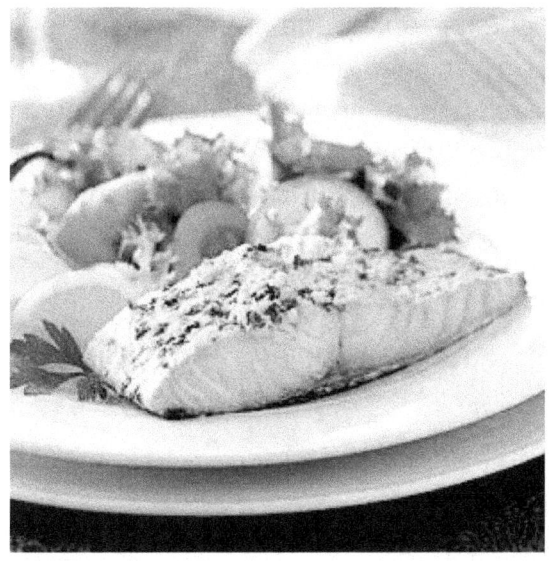

SERVINGS

4 persons

COOKING TIME

30 minutes

INGREDIENTS

Chopped fresh basil: 4 tbsp

Chopped fresh parsley: 1 tbsp

Minced garlic: 1 tbsp

Lemon juice: 2 tbsp

Salmon fillets: 4

Black pepper: to taste

Chopped olives: 4

Thin lemon slices: 4

PREPARATION METHOD

1. Spray the grill with cooking spray and heat the grill.
2. Combine basil, parsley, minced garlic, and lemon juice in a small bowl.
3. Sprinkle fish with black pepper and coat with basil-garlic mixture.
4. Grill the fish over high heat for 3 minutes on each side.
5. Serve warm garnished with green olives and lemon slices.

NUTRITION VALUE PER SERVING

Calories: 183

Fat: 9g

Protein: 30g

Carbohydrates: 10g

Buffalo and Turkey Chili

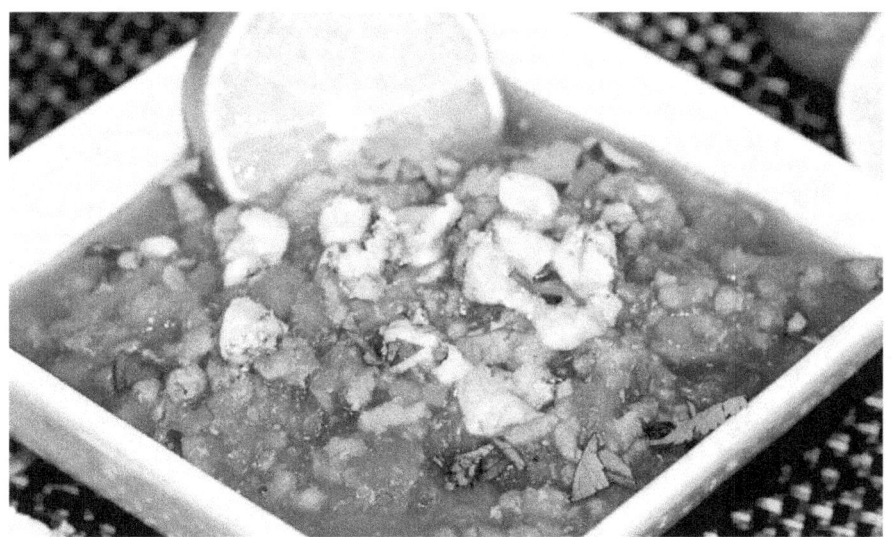

SERVINGS

2 persons

COOKING TIME

1 hour

INGREDIENTS

Lean ground buffalo meat: 1 pound

Lean ground turkey: 1 pound

Chopped onions: 2

Chopped celery stalks: 3

Minced garlic cloves: 2

Fire-roasted tomatoes: 114 oz can

Strained tomatoes: 4 cups

Low-sodium chicken broth: 5 cups

Chopped zucchini: 3

Chopped bell pepper: 1

Red quinoa: 2 cups

Smoked sweet paprika: 1 tbsp

Cinnamon: 2 tsp

Butter: 1 tbsp

Grated cheddar cheese: ½ cup

Salt

Pepper

PREPARATION METHOD

1. Melt butter over medium heat and add onion and garlic. Cook for about 3 minutes and add carrots and celery. Cook until soft.
2. Cook the buffalo and turkey meat for about 5 minutes over medium-high heat.
3. Add tomatoes, paprika, cinnamon, sea salt, and pepper. Add the chicken broth slowly and bring to simmer. Cook over low heat for 60 to 70 minutes.
4. Prepare quinoa and set aside.
5. Season zucchini with sea salt and pepper. Grill over medium high heat until cooked.
6. Serve with red bell pepper and cheddar cheese, topped with quinoa, zucchini, and cheese.

NUTRITION VALUE PER SERVING

Calories: 330

Fat: 8.5g

Protein: 32.6g

Carbohydrates: 31.6g

Butternut Squash Frittata

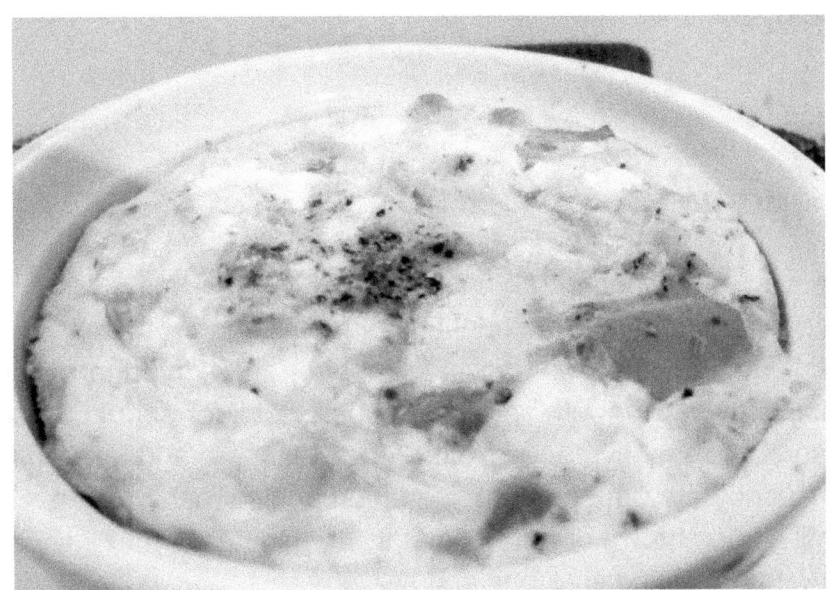

SERVINGS

6 persons

COOKING TIME

20 minutes

INGREDIENTS

Thinly sliced Japanese eggplant: 2

Chopped red onion: 1

Chopped cremini mushrooms: 8 oz

Cubed butternut squash: 12 oz.

Diced scallions: 5

Sprigs thyme: 5

Eggs: 6

Butter: 1 tbsp

Extra virgin coconut oil: 1 tbsp

Sea salt

Pepper

PREPARATION METHOD

1. Preheat oven to 350 degrees F
2. Grill the eggplant on both sides until brown, seasoned with salt.
3. Over medium-high heat, cook onion with butter and add butternut squash after 3 minutes. Lightly season with salt and pepper. Cook for about 6 minutes and then add mushrooms and thyme. Cook for 3 minutes more and take off from heat.
4. Layer a baking tray with eggplant and onion and squash mixture.
5. Bake until golden brown or approximately 20 minutes.
6. Garnish with remaining scallions and serve hot.

NUTRITION VALUE PER SERVING

Calories: 160

Fat: 9.5g

Protein: 8.7g

Carbohydrates: 12.8g

Chicken Kebabs with Spicy Carrot Tahini

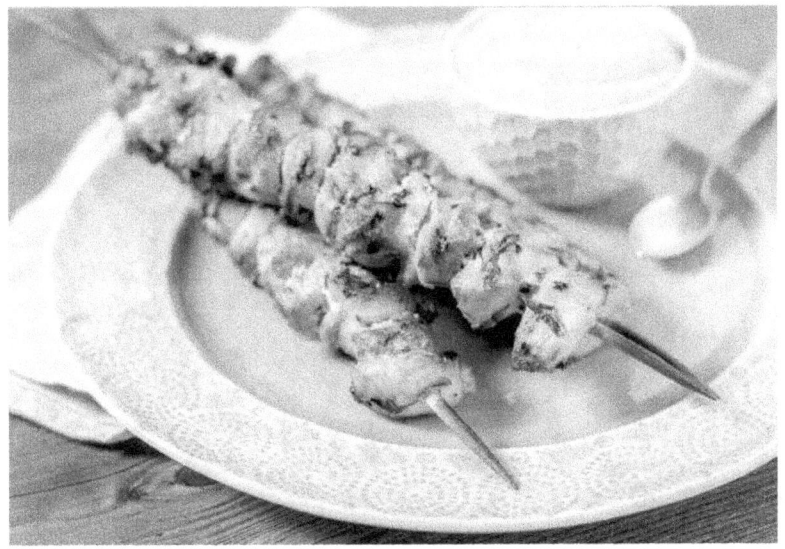

SERVINGS

6 persons

COOKING TIME

25-30 minutes

INGREDIENTS

Chicken breast: 2 ½ lbs

Extra virgin coconut oil: 3 tbsp

Chopped oregano: 1 tbsp

Chopped basil: 1tbsp

Sea salt: ½ tsp

To Make Spicy Tahini:

Peeled and sliced carrots: 4-6

Coconut oil: 1 tbsp (for pan)

Smashed garlic cloves: 3

Extra virgin coconut oil: ¼ cup

Water: 1 ½ cup

Juiced lemon: ½

Tahini: ½ cup

Sea salt: 1 tsp

Cayenne: ½ tsp

PREPARATION METHOD

1. Preheat grill.
2. Place cubes of chicken breast in a mixing bowl. Add 3 tbsp extra virgin coconut oil, oregano, basil, and salt. Mix well and let it sit.
3. Cook the sliced carrots in light coconut oil for about 10-12 minutes or until edges are brown.
4. Grill the chicken cubes while carrots are cooking.
5. Blend the carrots in a food processor once they are cooked. Cook garlic for 30 seconds or until brown, add with coconut oil, water, and lemon juice to food processor, and blend until smooth. Pour tahini, cayenne pepper and salt (to taste) to blend in with the mixture.
6. Serve the hot chicken kebabs with spicy tahini sauce and enjoy!

NUTRITION VALUE PER SERVING

Calories: 373

Fat: 13.8g

Protein: 60.8g

Carbohydrates: 0.5g

Pasta with Mediterranean Twist

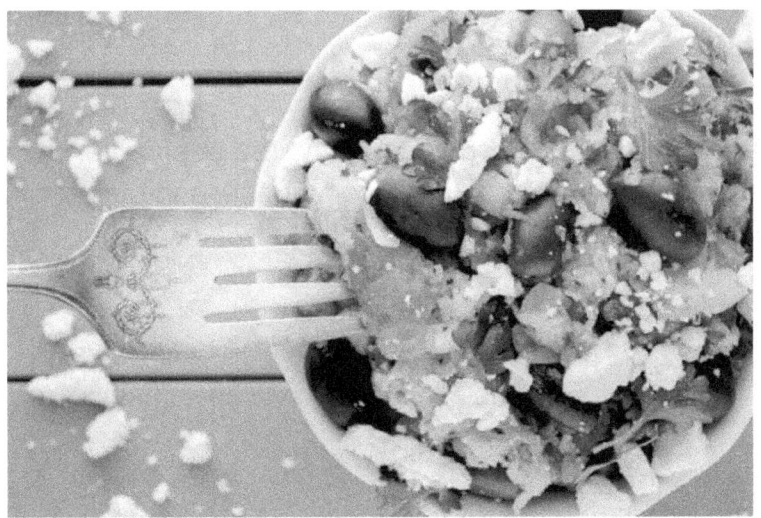

SERVINGS

4 persons

COOKING TIME

25 minutes

INGREDIENTS

Zucchini: 4

Garlic clove: 1

Drained and rinsed capers: 2 tbsp

Crushed red pepper flakes: ¼ tsp

Extra virgin coconut oil: 2 tbsp

Drained and diced tomatoes: 1 can

Finely chopped kalamata olives: ½ cup

Grass-fed butter: 2 tbsp

Chopped basil: 3 tbsp

PREPARATION METHOD

1. Slice the zucchini and sprinkle with salt.
2. Make a paste with garlic, 1 tbsp capers, and red pepper flakes.
3. Add the paste with remaining capers, coconut oil, and tomatoes to a mixing bowl.
4. Sauté zucchini in butter for 3 minutes and toss with sauce
5. Serve with fresh basil.

NUTRITION VALUE PER SERVING

Calories: 151

Fat: 9.6g

Protein: 5.1g

Carbohydrates: 16.1g

Red Lentil Soup

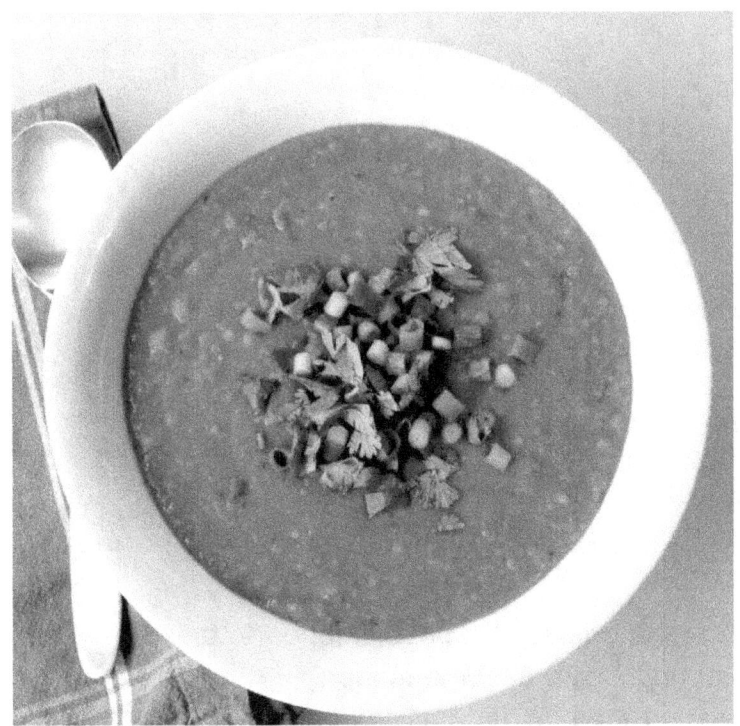

SERVINGS

4 persons

COOKING TIME

1 hour 15 minutes

INGREDIENTS

Coconut oil: 2 tbsp

Chopped onion: 1

Ground cumin: 1 tsp

Ground coriander: ½ tsp

Red pepper flakes: a pinch

Rinsed and split red lentils: 1 cup

Peeled and chopped carrot: 1

Peeled and chopped tomato: 1

Vegetable stock: 4 cups

Salt

Pepper

Lemon juice: 2 tbsp

PREPARATION METHOD

1. Heat coconut oil over medium heat in a large pot. Sauté onion and cook for 5 minutes until soft. Stir cumin, coriander, and red pepper flakes and cook for 5 minutes.
2. Add lentils, carrot, tomato, stick, salt, pepper (to taste), and bring to boil. Cook for 40 minutes or until lentils become tender.
3. Process the soup in a blender until smooth.
4. Serve hot with lemon juice.

NUTRITION VALUE PER SERVING

Calories: 194

Fat: 7g

Protein: 11g

Carbohydrates: 23g

Gazpacho

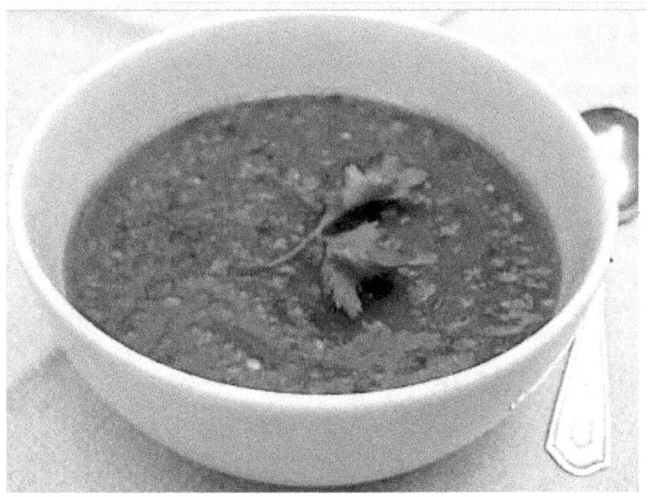

SERVINGS

4 persons

COOKING TIME

10-15 minutes

INGREDIENTS

Fresh tomatoes: 2 lb

Chopped garlic cloves: 2

Diced tomatoes: 1 can

Peeled and chopped cucumber: 1

Chopped red onion: ½

Chopped red pepper: 1

Vinegar: 1 tbsp

Coconut oil: 2 tsp

Salt

Pepper

PREPARATION METHOD

1. Combine tomatoes and garlic in blender and process to a coarse puree.
2. Add all ingredients except salt and pepper and blend until smooth.
3. Refrigerate, and serve chilled topped with salt and pepper to taste, and garnished with cucumber and onions if desired.

NUTRITION VALUE PER SERVING

Calories: 91

Fat: 1g

Protein: 4g

Carbohydrates: 20g

Chicken and Seafood Paella

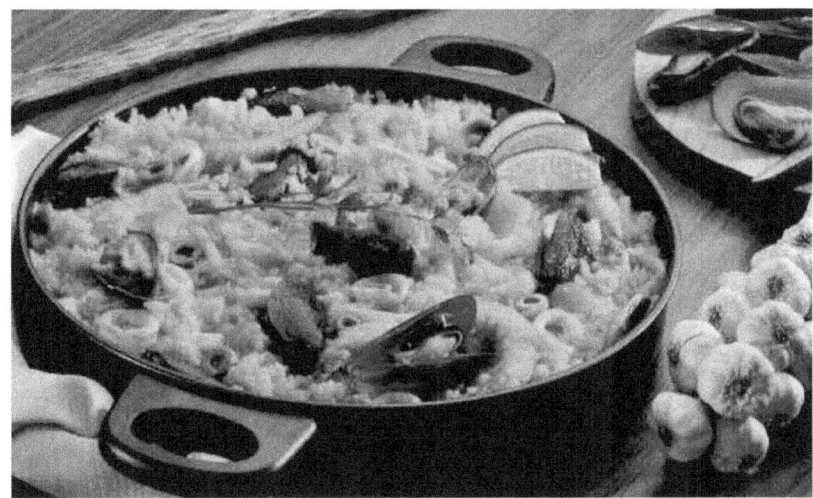

SERVINGS

4 persons

COOKING TIME

30 minutes

INGREDIENTS

Saffron: ¼ tsp

Boneless chicken breast: 1 lb

Coconut oil: 2 tbsp

Sliced chorizo sausage: 6 oz

Chopped onion: 1

Minced garlic clove: 1

Pureed canned tomatoes: 2/3 cup

Chicken stock: 5 cups

Smoked paprika: 1 tsp

Scrubbed mussels: 12

Peeled and deveined shrimps: 12

Roasted red pepper: ½ cup

Thawed frozen peas: ½ cup

Lemon wedges: 3

PREPARATION METHOD

1. Toast saffron thread over medium heat for 1 minute. Put in small bowl and crush when cool.
2. Heat oil in pan. Cook chorizo for about 2 minutes or until brown. Add chicken sprinkled with salt and pepper and cook until brown for about 5 minutes.
3. Remove chicken and add onion, garlic, and sauté until onion is soft. Add tomatoes, stock, paprika, and saffron, bring to boil and lower the heat
4. Add mussels and shrimp. Cook for another 10 minutes.
5. Add red pepper strips and peas after removing from heat and let it stand for 10 minutes.
6. Serve hot garnished with lemon wedges.

NUTRITION VALUE PER SERVING

Calories: 319

Fat: 14g

Protein: 28g

Carbohydrates: 18g

ALADS

Chopped Greek Salad

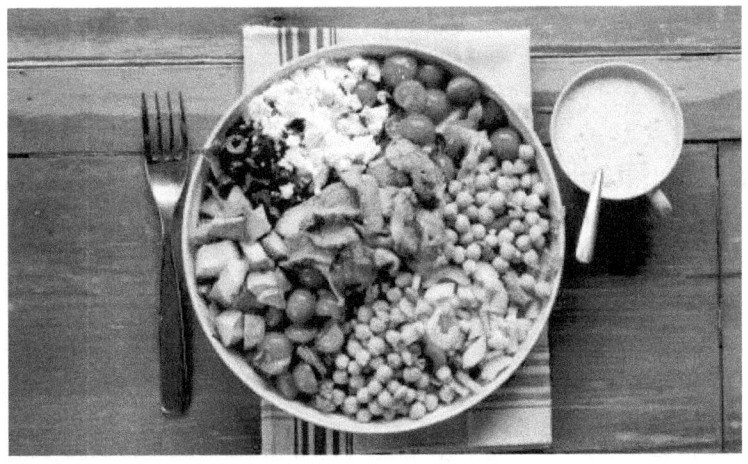

SERVINGS

1-2 persons

COOKING TIME

10 minutes

INGREDIENTS

Sliced cucumber: 1

Green onion: 2

Cherry or grape tomatoes: 1 pint

Kalamata olives: 1 handful

Pepperoncini peppers: 4

Arugula greens: 2 handfuls

Lemon juice: 1 tbsp

Red wine vinegar: 2 tbsp

Extra virgin coconut oil: 3 tbsp

Salt

Pepper

PREPARATION METHOD

1. Chop the cucumber, green onions, tomatoes, olives, peppers, and arugula.
2. Toss them into a bowl with everything else and mix well.
3. Season salad with salt and pepper generously before serving.

NUTRITION VALUE PER SERVING

Calories: 380

Fat: 30g

Protein: 3g

Carbohydrates: 15g

Mediterranean Tuna Salad

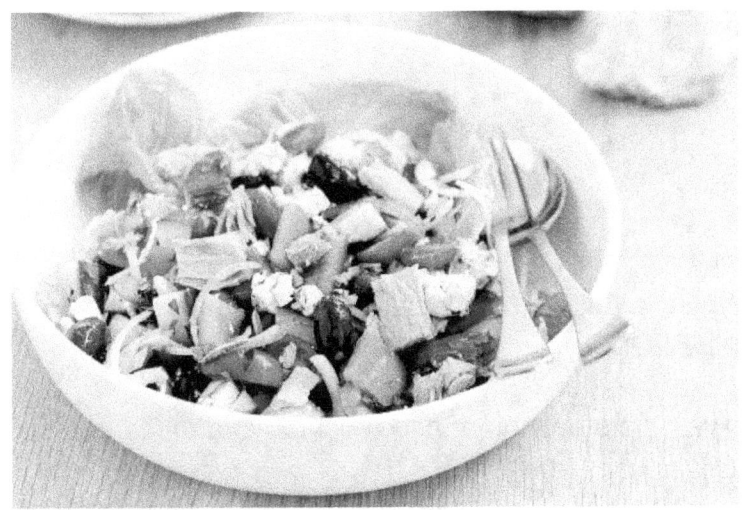

SERVINGS

2 persons

COOKING TIME

10-20 minutes

INGREDIENTS

White albacore tuna: 1 can

Kalamata olives: 10

Roughly chopped parsley: 1 tbsp

Roughly chopped, quartered artichokes: 1 can

For Dressing

Mayonnaise: 1 tbsp

Coconut oil: a drizzle

Lemon juiced: ½

Garlic powder: ¼ tsp

Red pepper flakes: 1/8 tsp

Oregano: ¼ tsp

Salt

Pepper

PREPARATION METHOD

1. Mix tuna, olives, parsley, onion, and artichokes in medium sized bowl and drizzle with coconut oil.
2. In another bowl, add mayo, lemon juice, garlic powder, red pepper flakes, oregano, salt, and pepper and whisk to combine well.
3. Pour dressing over tuna mixture and stir.
4. Serve chilled.

NUTRITION VALUE PER SERVING

Calories: 34

Fat: 2.4g

Protein: 0.4g

Carbohydrates: 3.2g

Chinese Chicken Salad

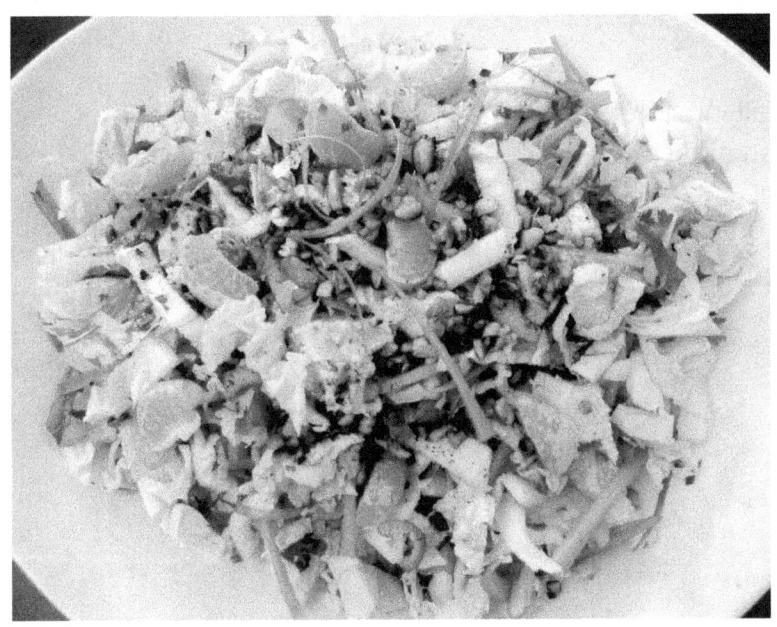

SERVINGS

2 persons

COOKING TIME

10 minutes

INGREDIENTS

Fine shredded cabbage: 4 cups

Carrot: 1 cup

Scallions: ¼ cup

Radishes: ¼ cup

Chopped cilantro: ¼ cup

Fresh mint: ¼ cup

Cooked chicken: 2 cups

PREPARATION METHOD

1. Combine all ingredients and mix well.
2. Serve fresh and refrigerated with a salad dressing of your choice, or you can also have it plain.

NUTRITION VALUE PER SERVING

Calories: 67

Fat: 0.4g

Protein: 3.9g

Carbohydrates: 14.7g

Grapes, Feta and Mint Salad

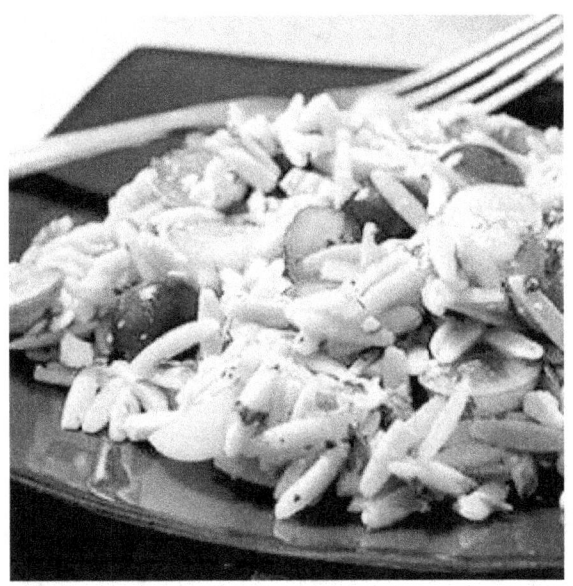

SERVINGS

4 persons

COOKING TIME

30-40 minutes

INGREDIENTS

Water: 1 ½ cup

Bulgur wheat: 1 cup

Fresh lemon juice: ¼ cup

Coconut oil: 1 tbsp

Salt: ½ tsp

Ground cumin: ½ tsp

Cayenne pepper: a pinch

Diced seedless cucumber: 1 cup

Halved seedless grapes: ¾ cup

Crumbled fat-free feta: ½ cup

Chopped fresh mint: ¼ cup

Sliced scallions: 3 tbsp

PREPARATION METHOD

1. Boil water in a small saucepan and stir in bulgur. Remove from heat, cover pan and let it sit for 25-30 minutes until bulgur is tender.
2. In a large serving bowl, pour bulgur and add lemon juice, coconut oil, cumin, and cayenne.
3. After it cools, add cucumber, grapes, feta, mint, and scallions. Mix well.
4. Refrigerate and it is ready to serve.

NUTRITION VALUE PER SERVING

Calories: 195

Fat: 4g

Protein: 8g

Carbohydrates: 35g

Kale Crunch Salad

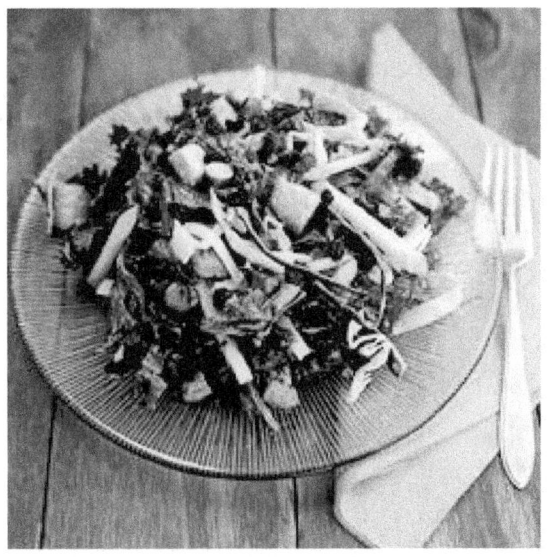

SERVINGS

1-2 persons

COOKING TIME

10 minutes

INGREDIENTS

Medium bunch kale: 1

Carrot: 1

Golden beets: ½ cup

Lemon juice: 1-2 lemons

Coconut oil: 1 tbsp

Salt

Pepper

Chopped nuts: ¼ cup

PREPARATION METHOD

1. Place thinly cut kale leaves into a bowl and add julienned carrot, beets, lemon juice, coconut oil, salt and pepper.
2. Stir thoroughly to combine and allow the salad to rest for at least 30 minutes for best results.
3. Serve topped with crushed nuts for a delicious crunch.

NUTRITION VALUE PER SERVING

Calories: 348

Fat: 31.8

Protein: 6.5g

Carbohydrates: 14.6g

Strawberry and Macadamia Nut Chicken Salad

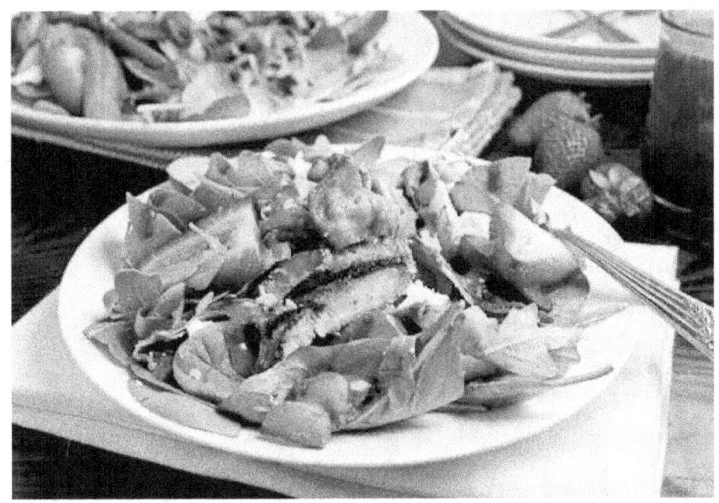

SERVINGS

3-4 persons

COOKING TIME

35-40 minutes

INGREDIENTS

Chicken breast: 1lb

Macadamia nut oil: 1 tsp

Salt and pepper: to taste

Chopped strawberries: 2 cups

Diced celery: ½ cup

Mayonnaise: 2 tbsp

Julienned basil: 2 tbsp

Lemon juice: 1 tbsp

PREPARATION METHOD

1. Bake chicken breast for about 35 minutes with a drizzle of oil, salt and pepper.
2. Shred chicken into a bowl and add, strawberries, nuts, celery, basil, mayo, lemon juice.
3. Stir and combine well.

NUTRITION VALUE PER SERVING

Calories: 380

Fat: 23g

Protein: 14g

Carbohydrates: 12g

Mexican Salad

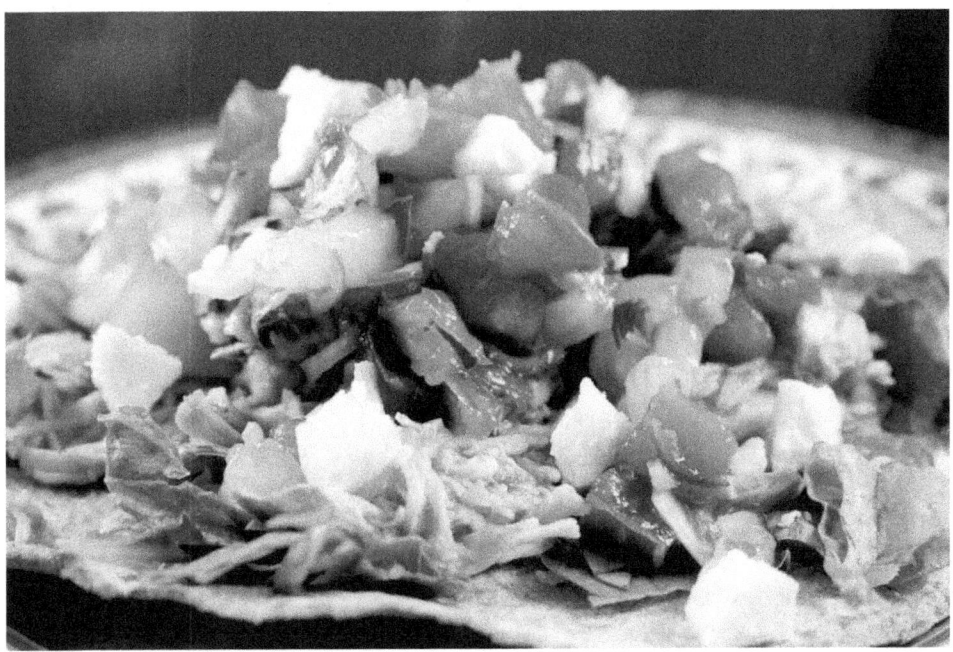

SERVINGS

3-4 persons

COOKING TIME

60 minutes

INGREDIENTS

For Chicken

Boneless chicken breast: 1lb

Coconut oil: 1 tbsp

Salt and pepper: to taste

For Salsa

Quartered tomato: 1

Red onion: ½ (cut into chunks)

Jalapeno pepper: 1

Peeled garlic clove: 1

Bunch of cilantro leaves: 1

Juiced lemon: 1

Salt and pepper: to taste

PREPARATION METHOD

1. Bake chicken breast brushed with oil, salt and pepper for about 35 minutes.
2. Meanwhile, blend all salsa ingredients in food processor. Shred chicken pieces after it is cool.
3. Mix both ingredients well with a fork
4. Serve chilled or as you desire.

NUTRITION VALUE PER SERVING

Calories: 262

Fat: 12g

Protein: 33.4g

Carbohydrates: 3.5g

Basil Avocado Chicken Salad

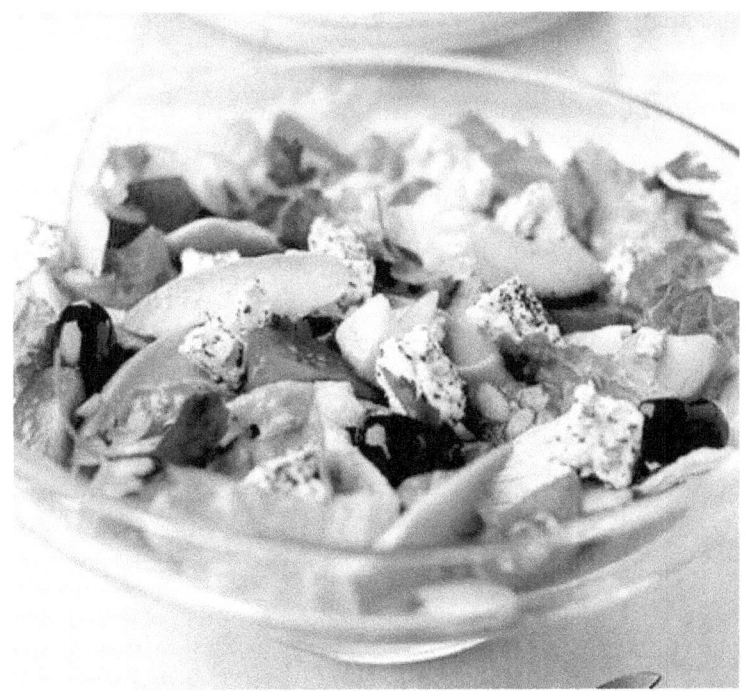

SERVINGS

2 persons

COOKING TIME

15 minutes

INGREDIENTS

Boneless chicken breasts: 2

Fresh basil leaves: ½ cup

Avocado: 1 large

Extra virgin coconut oil: 2 tbsp

Sea salt: ½ tsp

Ground black pepper: 1/8 tsp

PREPARATION METHOD

1. Blend basil, avocado, coconut oil, sea salt and ground pepper in food processor until smooth.
2. Shred the cooked chicken and mix it well with the avocado and basil mixture.
3. Refrigerate until ready to serve.

NUTRITION VALUE PER SERVING

Calories: 65

Fat: 7.1g

Protein: 8g

Carbohydrates: 5g

Broccoli Salad

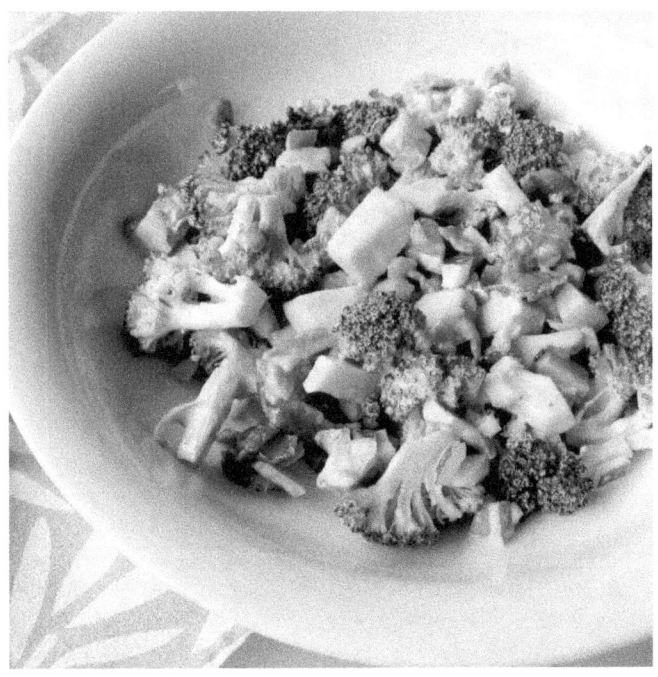

SERVINGS

3-4 persons

COOKING TIME

25-30 minutes

INGREDIENTS

Broccoli: 1lb

Chopped almonds: ¾ cup

Raisins: ½ cup

Bacon: 6 slices

Coconut oil: ½ cup

Apple cider vinegar: ¼ cup

Salt and pepper: to taste

PREPARATION METHOD

1. Bake bacon slices at 375 degree F or until brown and crispy, about 25 minutes.
2. Chop broccoli into pieces and add to bowl with vinegar, almonds, raisins, salt and pepper.
3. Chop bacon when cool and add to bowl with coconut oil.
4. Toss well to combine and serve.

NUTRITION VALUE PER SERVING

Calories: 208

Fat: 9.4g

Protein: 7.6g

Carbohydrates: 26.1g

Fruit Cinnamon Salad

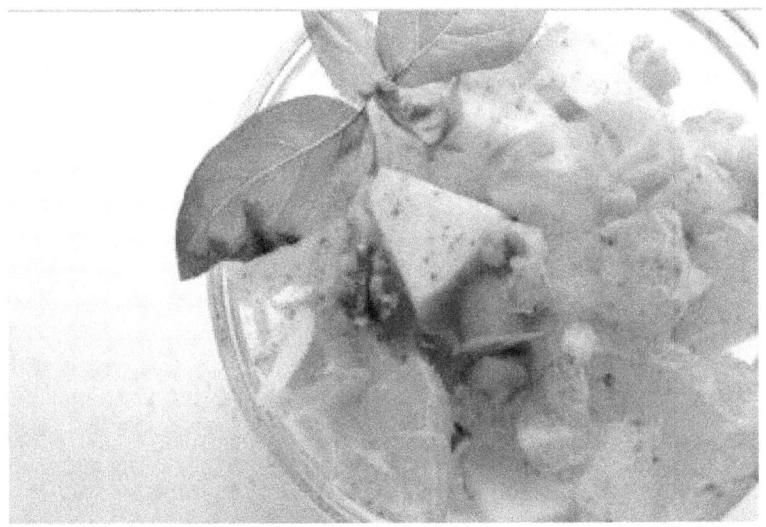

SERVINGS

1-2 persons

COOKING TIME

15 minutes

INGREDIENTS

Peeled and diced orange: 1

Diced apple: 1

Chopped walnuts: ½ cup

Cinnamon: ½ tsp

PREPARATION METHOD

1. Mix fruit in bowl
2. Serve with chopped nuts and cinnamon on top

NUTRITION VALUE PER SERVING

Calories: 184

Fat: 0.2g

Protein: 1.8g

Carbohydrates: 47.7g

Bean Salad

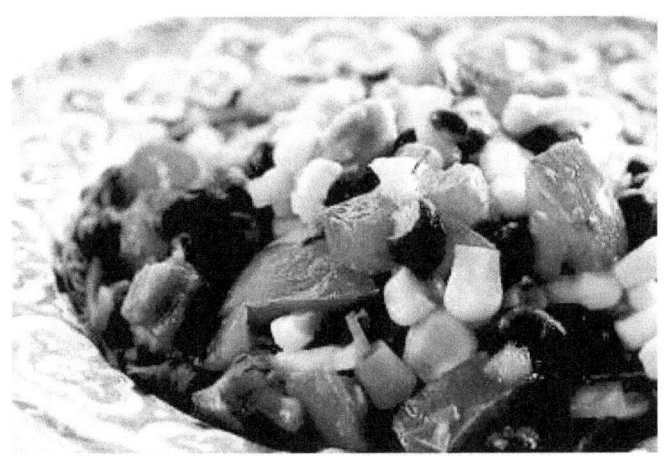

SERVINGS

6-8 persons

COOKING TIME

20-30 minutes

INGREDIENTS

Tender crisp cooked green beans: ¼ pound

Tender crisp cooked yellow beans: ¼ pound

Tender cooked black beans: 1 ½ cup

Tender cooked kidney-beans: 1 ½ cup

Sliced red onion: 1

Bell pepper: 1

Chopped celery stalk: 1

Salt and pepper: to taste

For Dressing

Honey: 1 cup

Cider vinegar: 1 cup

Vegetable oil: 1 cup

Tallow mustard: 1 cup

Salt: 1 ½ tsp

Celery seeds: 1 ½ tsp

PREPARATION METHOD

1. Prepare the dressing by mixing honey and vinegar in a tight jar. Shake well and let it stand for 15 minutes. Make sure the sugar dissolves in vinegar. Add remaining ingredients and mix well.
2. Mix veggies and beans in a bowl. Add dressing salt and pepper. Mix well.
3. Refrigerate until ready to serve.

NUTRITION VALUE PER SERVING

Calories: 130

Fat: 9.2g

Protein: 6g

Carbohydrates: 8g

Avocado and Roasted Asparagus Salad

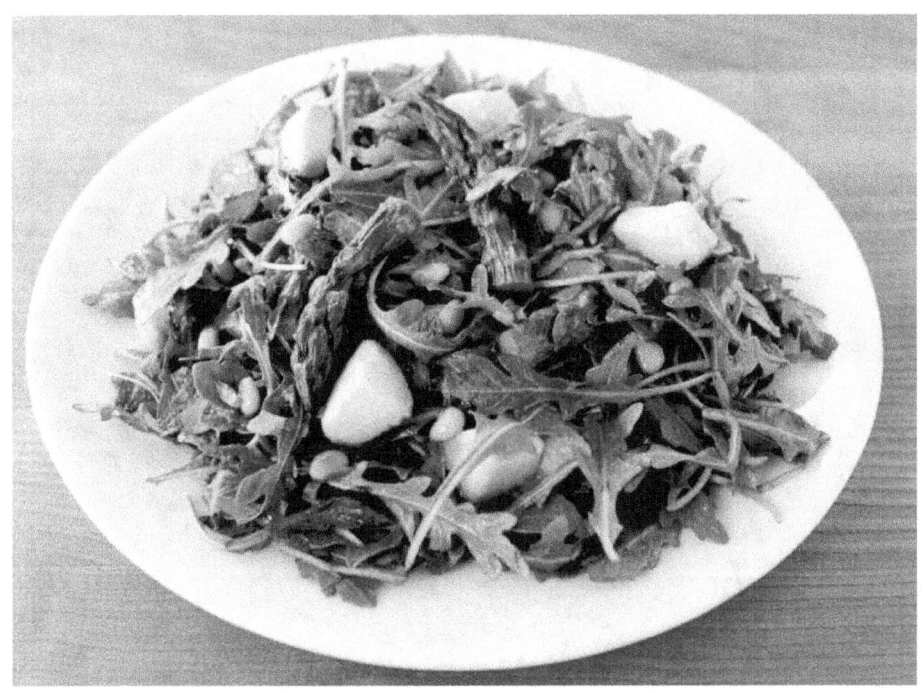

SERVINGS

4 persons

COOKING TIME

15-20 minutes

INGREDIENTS

Asparagus: 1 lb

Coconut oil: 1 tbsp

Sea salt: to taste

Spring mix salad greens: 5 ounces

Thinly sliced red onions: ½

Grape tomatoes: 1 cup

Sliced avocado: 1

To make lemon garlic vinaigrette

Lemon juice: ¼ cup

Minced garlic clove: 1

Dijon mustard: 1 tbsp

Red pepper flakes: 1/8 tsp

Extra-virgin coconut oil: ¼ cup

Sea salt: to taste

PREPARATION METHOD

1. Prepare the vinaigrette by mixing all ingredients. Stir well and set aside.
2. Pre heat oven to 400 degree F and roast asparagus, sprinkled with sea salt and with a drizzle of coconut oil for 10-15 minutes or until crisp tender.
3. Arrange salad greens in plates. Top with roasted asparagus, tomatoes, onion and avocado.
4. Serve with the vinaigrette.

NUTRITION VALUE PER SERVING

Calories: 260

Fat: 3g

Protein: 5g

Carbohydrates: 13g

Turkey Salad with Potato Fries

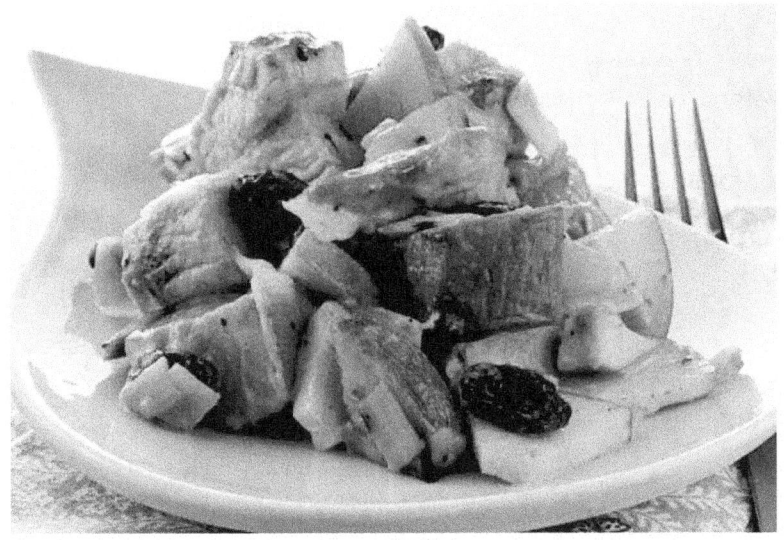

SERVINGS

6 persons

COOKING TIME

20-30 minutes

INGREDIENTS

For Potato Fries:

Sweet potatoes: 2

Coconut oil: 4 tbsp

Finely chopped sage leaves: 4 tsp

Sea salt and pepper

For Dressing

Balsamic vinegar: 3 tbsp

Extra virgin coconut oil: 1/3 cup

Cranberry juice: 1/3 cup

Dijon mustard: 1 ½ tsp

Orange zest: 1 ½ tsp

Chopped green onions: 2

Salt and pepper

For Salad

Sliced romaine lettuce: 6 cups

Cooked turkey cubes: 2 cups

Sliced celery stalks: 2

Chopped pecans: ½ cup

Dried cranberries: ¼ cup

PREPARATION METHOD

1. Prepare the sweet potatoes by tossing with coconut oil, sage, salt and pepper to taste, in bowl. Bake for 20 minutes, turning once mid-way.
2. Meanwhile prepare the salad dressing by combining all ingredients and mix well.
3. Add the salad ingredients together in a bowl and serve with sweet potatoes and dressing.

NUTRITION VALUE PER SERVING

Calories: 300

Fat: 17g

Protein: 17g

Carbohydrates: 25g

Gingered Carrot and Date Salad

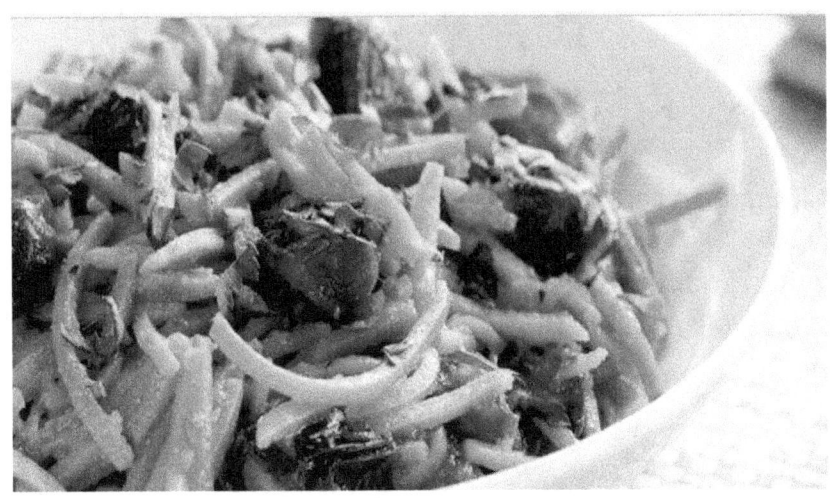

SERVINGS

4 persons

COOKING TIME

10-15 minutes

INGREDIENTS

Peeled and grated carrots: 1 pound

Chopped medjool dates: ½ cup

Coconut oil: 1 tbsp

Cider vinegar: 2 tbsp

Grated garlic cloves: 1

Honey: 1 tbsp

Cinnamon: ¼ tsp

Fresh grated ginger: 1 tsp

Salt: 1/8 tsp

Cayenne pepper: a pinch

Parsley: 1 tbsp

PREPARATION METHOD

1. Whisk oil, vinegar, garlic and sugar in large bowl and add cinnamon, ginger, salt and pepper.
2. Stir in carrots and refrigerate
3. Serve with parsley garnish.

NUTRITION VALUE PER SERVING

Calories: 160

Fat: 3.5g

Protein: 2g

Carbohydrates: 33g

Mediterranean Savory Salad

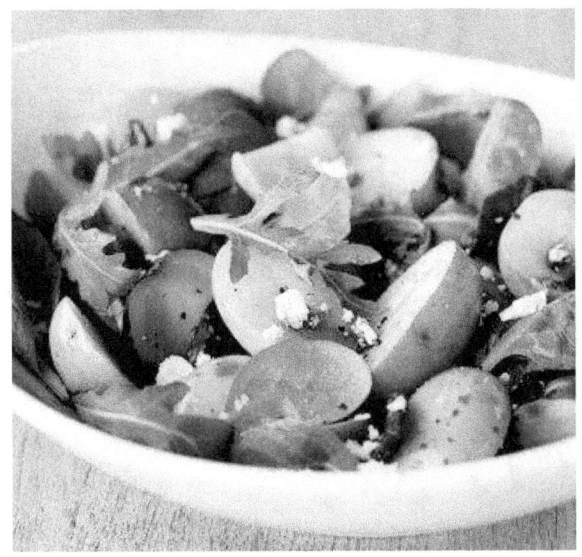

SERVINGS

6 persons

COOKING TIME

15-20 minutes

INGREDIENTS

Sweet potatoes: 3 pound

Chopped tomatoes: 4

Crumbled feta cheese: ¼ cup

Spinach: 5 cups

Balsamic vinegar: 2 tbsp

Extra virgin coconut oil: ¼ cup

Salt

Pepper

PREPARATION METHOD

1. Boil sweet potatoes until tender. Cut into pieces and add in bowl with other ingredients.
2. Mix all ingredients well and serve.

NUTRITION VALUE PER SERVING

Calories: 230

Fat: 8g

Protein: 5g

Carbohydrates: 0g